Bloody Powerful

Brilliantly illustrated with art from talented illustrator Hazel Mead, this incredible book is aimed at every woman stuck in the 'information gap' navigating the jargon and myths about their gynaecological health online.

Bloody Powerful covers everything you didn't get taught in school: giving you factually correct and reliable information coming from a practising gynaecology doctor. It is a non-judgemental and insightful guide to empowering yourself to take charge of your body. Dr Brooke Vandermolen answers questions you have always wanted to ask, from 'Do I need supplements to balance my hormones?' to 'How do I know if my period is too heavy?' sprinkled with facts you may never have realised about your body.

Thought-provoking, inspiring, and inclusive, this book will show you how we're all the same in wanting to know more about our own bodies, and we are each utterly and beautifully unique.

For many, **Dr Brooke Vandermolen** is better known by her online handle, 'The OBGYN Mum'. Brooke is a practising obstetrics and gynaecology doctor in London hospitals. She has a particular interest and experience in benign gynaecology with a focus on paediatric and adolescent gynaecology.

Brooke's journey into creating medical content as 'The OBGYN Mum' started with her first pregnancy. Despite her medical qualifications, Brooke found it difficult to obtain accurate, evidence-based information that she could understand and trust to guide her through her first pregnancy and parenthood. Alarmed at how much harder it would be for the average parent, Brooke decided to use her knowledge and credentials to create her platform 'The OBGYN Mum'.

To her rapidly growing audience, Brooke began sharing insights and tips around pregnancy, birth, fertility, menopause, and more through social media and blog posts. Her evidence-based information has since taken the internet by storm, smashing down taboos around areas of previously reserved areas of medicine.

Illustrator **Hazel Mead** uses her diverse, poignant art to discuss topics not explored enough, while inviting us all to look at each other with empathy. Her cute, playful style along with a sense of humour helps to soften some of the taboo topics she illustrates, making them a little more palatable for British sensibilities. She takes great joy in tugging on people's heartstrings and funny bones, which has resulted in a dedicated online following who resonates with her pieces. Hazel works commercially across publishing, advertising, branding, and mural painting. Her debut book *Why Aren't We Talking About This?!* was released by Squarepeg, Penguin last year.

'This is such an important book! Everything I wish I'd been taught at school, a must read!'

Hayley Morris, actor and author of *Me vs Brain: An Overthinker's Guide to Life*

'*Bloody Powerful* is a vital contribution to the growing movement to give women the information they deserve about their bodies. What makes this book stand out is Brooke's expertise, clarity and compassion which shine through every page.'

Dr Anita Mitra, gynaecologist and author of *The Gynae Geek*

'Halle-'bloody'-lujah! An accessible, entertaining and empowering book on the female experience. The topics are thoughtfully and thoroughly covered while the illustrations bring an empowered, light-hearted vibe. Normalising and taboo-smashing at its finest!'

Bex Gunn, co-founder of The Worst Girl Gang Ever Foundation and author of *The Worst Girl Gang Ever: A Survival Guide for Navigating Miscarriage and Pregnancy Loss*

'Empower yourself by reading this no-holds-barred guide to the cycles and complexities of the female body.'

Vanessa Feltz, broadcaster and presenter of 'Vanessa'

'Candid, clear, and anything but boring, this book tackles the subjects no one talks about – but every woman deserves to understand. A must-read from a voice you can trust.'

Sarah Jossel, journalist, broadcaster and beauty expert

'We all have questions, and it can be difficult to know where to go and who to trust to get the correct answers. This book makes it simple – if you have a question about women's health, Brooke has the answer! Buy it, borrow it from the library, share it with your friends, everyone needs the information in this book!'

Dr Philippa Kaye, GP, journalist and author of *The Science of Menopause: Understand Your Body, Make the Right Choices*

'This book is bloody brilliant. I wish I could have read it in my teens and twenties. Brooke tells it like it is, with humour and empathy.'

Dr Liz O'Riordan, author of *The Cancer Roadmap*

'*Bloody Powerful* is a bold, brilliant and much-needed guide that cuts through the noise and empowers women with clear, compassionate, and evidence-based information about their bodies. Brooke Vandermolen and Hazel Mead have created something truly special. A must-read for anyone navigating the complexities of gynaecological health.'

Jenny Halpern Prince MBE, co-founder of The Lady Garden Foundation

'Brooke has written the book that we wished we had growing up. Empowering, informative, insightful and accessible – this will change the way girls, and women, understand themselves and their bodies going forward. An ally for every woman, from puberty to menopause and beyond.'

Samantha Silver and Gemma Rose Breger, co-founders of This is Mothership

PERIODS

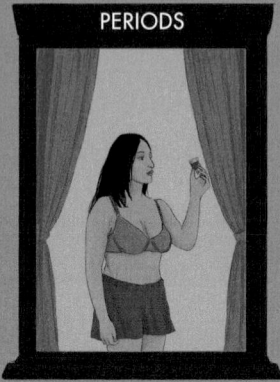

SEX

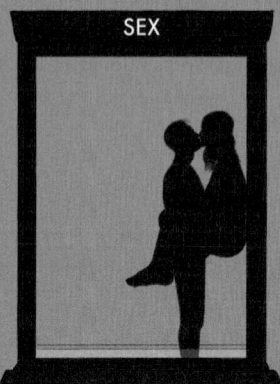

HORMONES

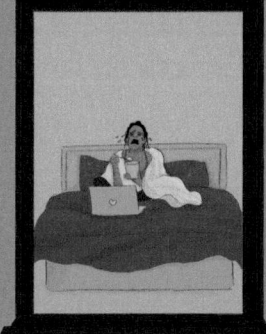

FERTILITY

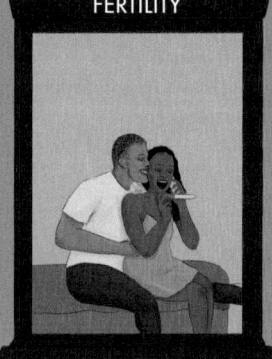

CONTRACEPTION

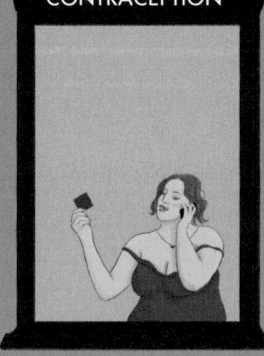

PREGNANCY

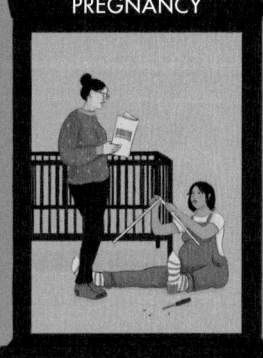

PREGNANCY LOSS

MENOPAUSE

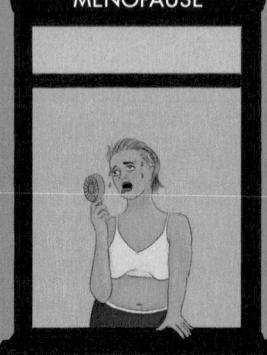

Bloody Powerful

The taboo-busting guide to periods, menopause and everything in-between

Dr Brooke Vandermolen
The OBGYN Mum

Illustrated by
Hazel Mead

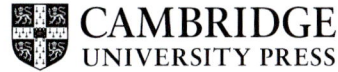

CAMBRIDGE
UNIVERSITY PRESS

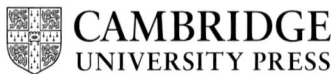

CAMBRIDGE
UNIVERSITY PRESS

Shaftesbury Road, Cambridge CB2 8EA, United Kingdom

One Liberty Plaza, 20th Floor, New York, NY 10006, USA

477 Williamstown Road, Port Melbourne, VIC 3207, Australia

314–321, 3rd Floor, Plot 3, Splendor Forum, Jasola District Centre,
  New Delhi – 110025, India

103 Penang Road, #05-06/07, Visioncrest Commercial, Singapore 238467

Cambridge University Press is part of Cambridge University Press & Assessment,
a department of the University of Cambridge.

We share the University's mission to contribute to society through the pursuit of
education, learning and research at the highest international levels of excellence.

www.cambridge.org
Information on this title: www.cambridge.org/9781009435482
DOI: 10.1017/9781009435499

When citing this work, please include a reference to the DOI
10.1017/9781009435499

First published 2026

A catalogue record for this publication is available from the British Library

*A Cataloging-in-Publication data record for this book is available from the Library
of Congress*

ISBN 978-1-009-43548-2 Hardback

Contents

For everyone who picked up this book looking to truly understand their body and how it works: this book is for you!

To my husband: the ultimate frame who always encourages me to chase my goals while building our family. This dream became a reality because of you!

And to my children, Lyla, Coby, and Jonah – my inspiration for everything. May your curiosity know no limits and never stop asking your endless questions.

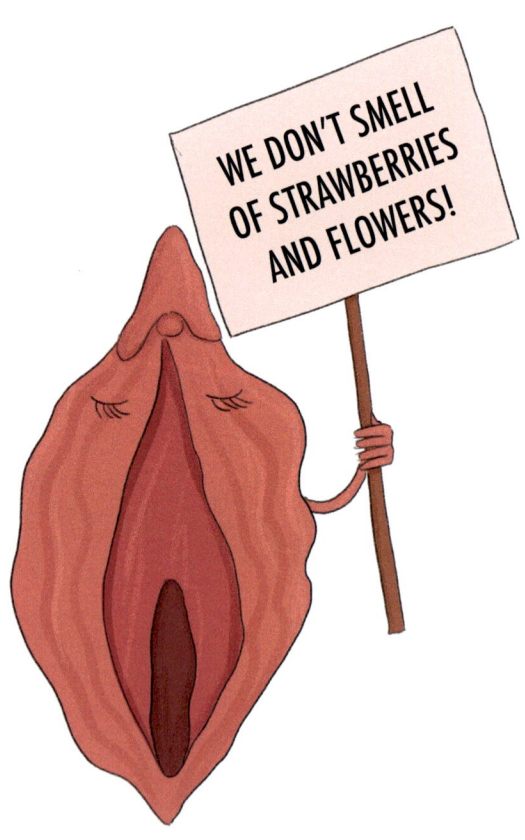

Introduction

Have you ever found yourself Googling, 'Is it safe to skip a period on the combined pill?' or scrolling through social media for answers to questions about how your body works? If so, you're not alone. Like many of you, my formal education on female health was pretty limited. School gave us the basics: a diagram of the reproductive system, a vague explanation of periods, and a not-so-subtle warning to avoid pregnancy. The deeper realities of female health – like what's actually happening during our cycles, why hormonal changes affect our moods, or how we can take control of our bodies – were largely ignored. It wasn't until I began working in obstetrics and gynaecology (O&G) that I realised just how much we aren't taught about our own bodies. I wanted to change that. I've seen just how much confusion there is about female health, and I knew there had to be a better way to share this information.

As a doctor training in O&G, I've spent years helping women navigate questions about their health. I've seen first-hand how little clear, reliable information is available, even when it comes to everyday concerns like painful periods, contraception options, or menopause symptoms. What I've also learned is that there's no *one-size-fits-all* when it comes to female health. Your body – and your health – are unique to you.

I wrote this book because I wanted you to read something that feels like a conversation with someone you trust – someone who has done the hard work of sifting through medical research, guidelines, and evidence to deliver answers you can rely on. This isn't a textbook full of jargon, and it's not just another opinion from the depths of the internet. It's a guide to help you understand what's going on with your body at every stage of life.

We'll talk about the things no one mentions – like how hormones influence your mood, why sex might feel different after menopause, and what you can do about those heavy, unpredictable periods. This book is here to answer your questions, demystify the science, and empower you to take control of your health. Your body doesn't come with an instruction manual – but if it did, I hope this would be it!

Before we dive deeper into the topics in this book, I want to briefly explain the interplay between hormones, gender identity, and biological sex. Understanding this relationship will help clarify the language I use throughout the book and why I sometimes refer to specific genders or biological terms when discussing certain aspects of health.

I want to acknowledge that this is a work in progress. I don't claim to have the perfect approach, and I am continually learning from people across different communities. My goal is to use language that feels appropriate to those it relates to, while ensuring no one feels excluded. I hope this book reflects an effort to present evidence-based information with thoughtfulness and inclusivity.

Biological sex: the blueprint of our bodies

Biological sex refers to the physical and physiological characteristics that include our reproductive organs, chromosomes, and hormones. As a gynaecologist, my focus often centres on the biological aspects of sex, particularly the intricate workings of the reproductive system traditionally classified as 'female'.

Biological sex is usually assigned at birth based on identifiable physical attributes, including the reproductive organs, hormones, and chromosomes. Those assigned female at birth generally have a vulva, with internal reproductive organs like ovaries and a uterus which may have been visible on an ultrasound. They typically produce higher levels of oestrogen and progesterone, and after puberty those assigned female usually develop secondary sex characteristics such as the breasts and pubic and underarm hair. On a genetic level, typically we describe females as having XX chromosomes, and males as having XY chromosomes.

There are many people who are also considered as women but do not fit into this neatly defined category, because there are multiple differences that can occur during sex development. These people may be described as 'intersex' or having a 'difference of sexual development (DSD) condition'. This often involves having a different combination of chromosomes, such as XO, XXX, or XXY, but still have the physical attributes that lead them to have been assigned female at birth, such as a vulva. Some estimates suggest as many as 1.7% of the population have differences that may be consistent with intersex traits, although the true number of people who require medical intervention as a result of these differences is thought to be much lower, around 1 in 1,500 births.[1] Biological sex is therefore not always binary, as variations can result in different combinations of reproductive organs, hormone levels, or chromosomal patterns that do not fit typical 'male' or 'female' classifications.

Gender: beyond binary constructs

Next, we come to the more flexible and fluid concept of gender, which goes beyond the binary framework of male and female. Gender is a social construction, and is not based purely on physical characteristics. It is a complex interplay of biology, identity, and culture and encompasses the roles, behaviours, and expectations that a society considers to classify individuals.

Traditionally, we would classify individuals into men and women, but actually gender encompasses a wide range of identities, including but not limited to:

- **Cisgender:** Individuals whose gender identity matches the sex they were assigned at birth (e.g., a person assigned female at birth who identifies as a woman)
- **Transgender:** Individuals whose gender identity differs from the sex they were assigned at birth (e.g., a person assigned male at birth who identifies as a woman)
- **Non-binary:** People who do not exclusively identify as male or female. They may identify as both, neither (sometimes called agender), or somewhere along the gender spectrum
- **Genderqueer:** A similar term to non-binary, used by people who reject the idea of a fixed gender. Genderqueer individuals may identify with multiple genders, or beyond the gender binary
- **Genderfluid:** Individuals who experience shifts in their gender identity over time. Their gender may change from male to female, to non-binary, or other identities

Gender is deeply personal and can be fluid, with people experiencing and expressing their gender in ways that are unique to them. Gender does not have a scientific definition, but rather it reflects how individuals perceive themselves and how they want to express their identity in relation to societal expectations.

As a gynaecologist, it's essential to acknowledge and respect our patients' diverse gender identities. This inclusive approach fosters a supportive environment for individuals of all genders to receive personalised and sensitive healthcare.

Gender dysphoria

Gender dysphoria is a psychological term that refers to the distress or discomfort that may occur when the gender someone is assigned at birth (based on their physical and physiological characteristics) does not align with their view of their own gender identity. In other words, it is the emotional and psychological distress that arises from the incongruence between one's assigned gender and their true gender identity. Individuals experiencing gender dysphoria may feel a strong desire to live and be recognised as a gender different from the one assigned to them at birth. One may choose to embrace and explore these feelings, or this distress can manifest in various ways, such as anxiety, depression, or a strong sense of unease with one's own body.

It's important to note that being transgender is not a mental health disorder. Many transgender individuals do not experience psychological distress or discomfort, especially if they are able to live in a way that aligns with their gender identity.

Medical and mental health professionals may work with individuals experiencing gender dysphoria to explore ways to alleviate the distress. This can involve social, psychological, and sometimes medical interventions, such as hormone therapy or gender-affirming surgeries, depending on the individual's needs and preferences. Understanding and respecting an individual's gender identity and providing appropriate support are crucial elements in addressing gender dysphoria and promoting mental well-being.

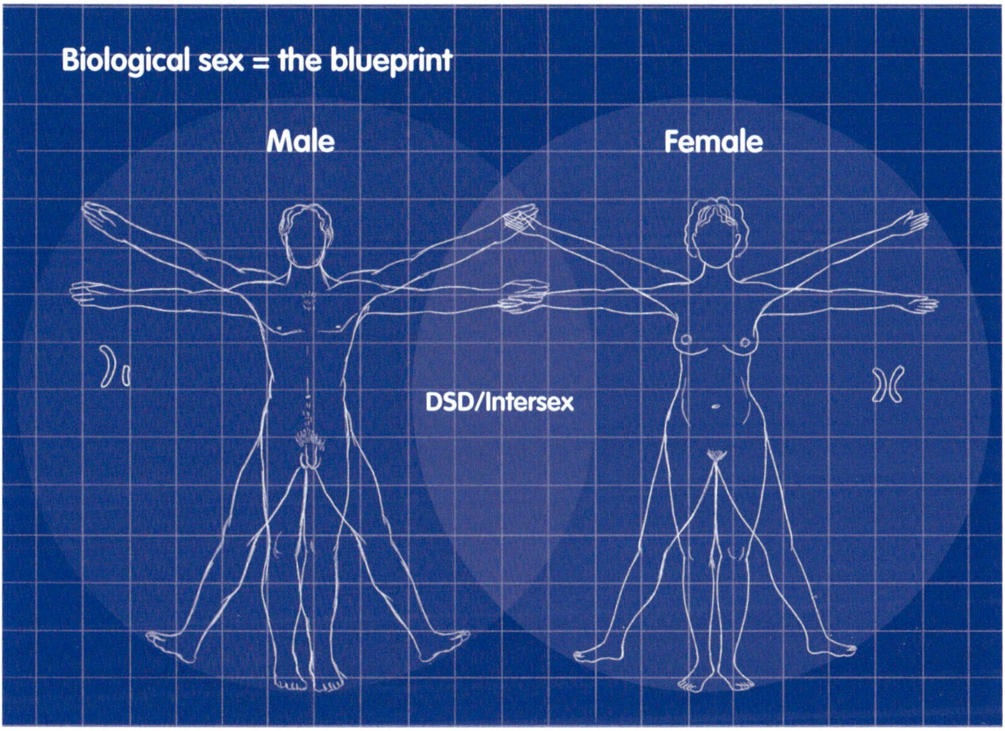

Biological sex = the blueprint

Male

Female

DSD/Intersex

Gender identity:

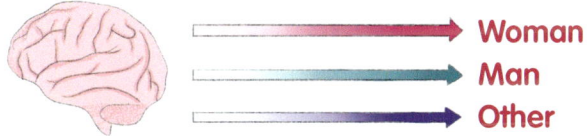

→ Woman
→ Man
→ Other

Gender expression:

Pronouns: he/him/she/her/they/them

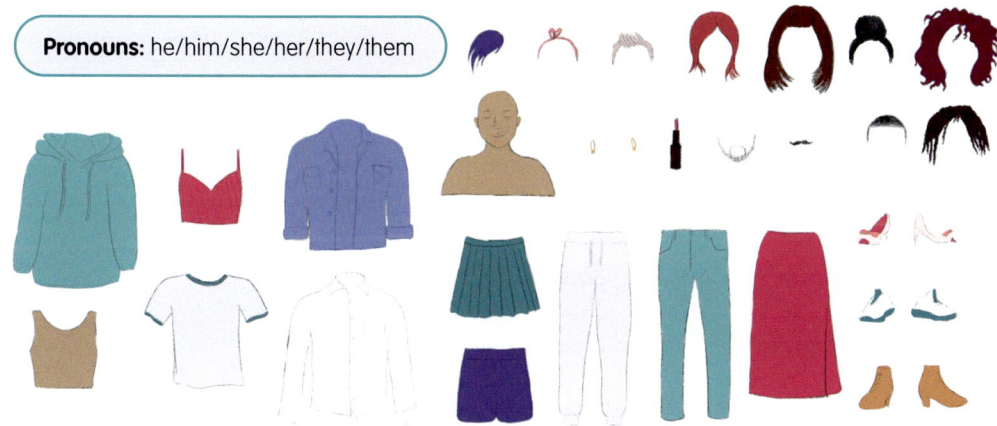

Intersectionality of sex and gender in healthcare

Recognising the intersectionality of sex and gender is crucial in providing comprehensive healthcare. For instance, transgender and non-binary individuals may have unique healthcare needs that extend beyond traditional models designed for cisgender individuals.

In my practice, I strive to provide care that places the patient at the centre, rather than what guidelines and protocols dictate, respecting the diverse identities and experiences of individuals. Ever since I started writing on social media, I have been working hard to eliminate any of my own internal bias that makes me assume other families are like mine.

In this book, you'll notice that I use terms like 'women', 'females', and 'people' interchangeably. This deliberate choice reflects the diverse groups I aim to include, recognising that no single term can encompass everyone's experiences. While gynaecology has traditionally been called a 'women's health' specialty, not everyone with a uterus or ovaries identifies as a woman. However, this inclusivity doesn't mean erasing the word 'woman'; instead, it's about ensuring everyone feels seen and respected.

Although transgender individuals make up a smaller percentage of the population, they often face significant marginalisation, including higher risks of medical discrimination, poverty, and violence. Similarly, many people identify as non-binary or come from family structures that differ from the traditional 'husband and wife' model, highlighting the need for inclusive language and approaches in healthcare.

I believe by expanding how we refer to people, we can help more people to feel seen and to feel included, ultimately encouraging them to engage with healthcare services when they need to. It is possible to advocate for all of these groups. We don't need to delete the word 'woman' or 'mother' from our vocabulary, instead I prefer to use phrases like:

 Women and birthing people

 Pregnant people and their partners

 People who have periods, people with a uterus, people with ovaries

Language should be fluid; it doesn't need to be fixed. We can adjust the terms we use to those which suit the person in front of us. If I am talking to someone directly who I know identifies as a woman, I feel comfortable to call her a mother. I can talk about myself as a woman and my own internal challenges of being a working mother. These words still feature in day-to-day conversation. However, when approaching someone new or speaking more generally about medical topics, I do not make assumptions about who I am speaking to. For example, someone who is pregnant may be a surrogate and so would not consider themselves as the 'mother' of the child. Instead, she may prefer to be called a pregnant woman, or a pregnant person.

I feel passionately that at the same time as moving towards a society that is inclusive and empathetic to others, we also need to advocate and champion women's rights now more than ever. Even in the twenty-first century, huge barriers still exist that prevent equality between men and women. We live in a time where decisions about healthcare that predominantly affect women's bodies have become politicised. Across the world, in workplaces, we still struggle to close the gender pay gap and have to fight for adequate em-ployment rights such as maternity leave. The fight has to continue because behind closed doors, in individual households, a society where we do not speak up for women who are marginalised and hidden can allow domestic abuse to occur and continue unchecked.

Some may consider adding this extra nuance to the terms we use to describe men and women as going a step too far but, for me, healthcare is about reaching everyone equally. It means providing care without judgement or preconceptions. We can be inclusive without negating or excluding other groups.

As we move forward, let's embrace the diversity that exists within the tapestry of human identity, respecting the intricate interplay of biology, identity, and culture.

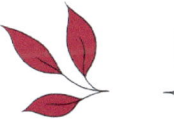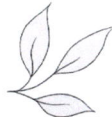

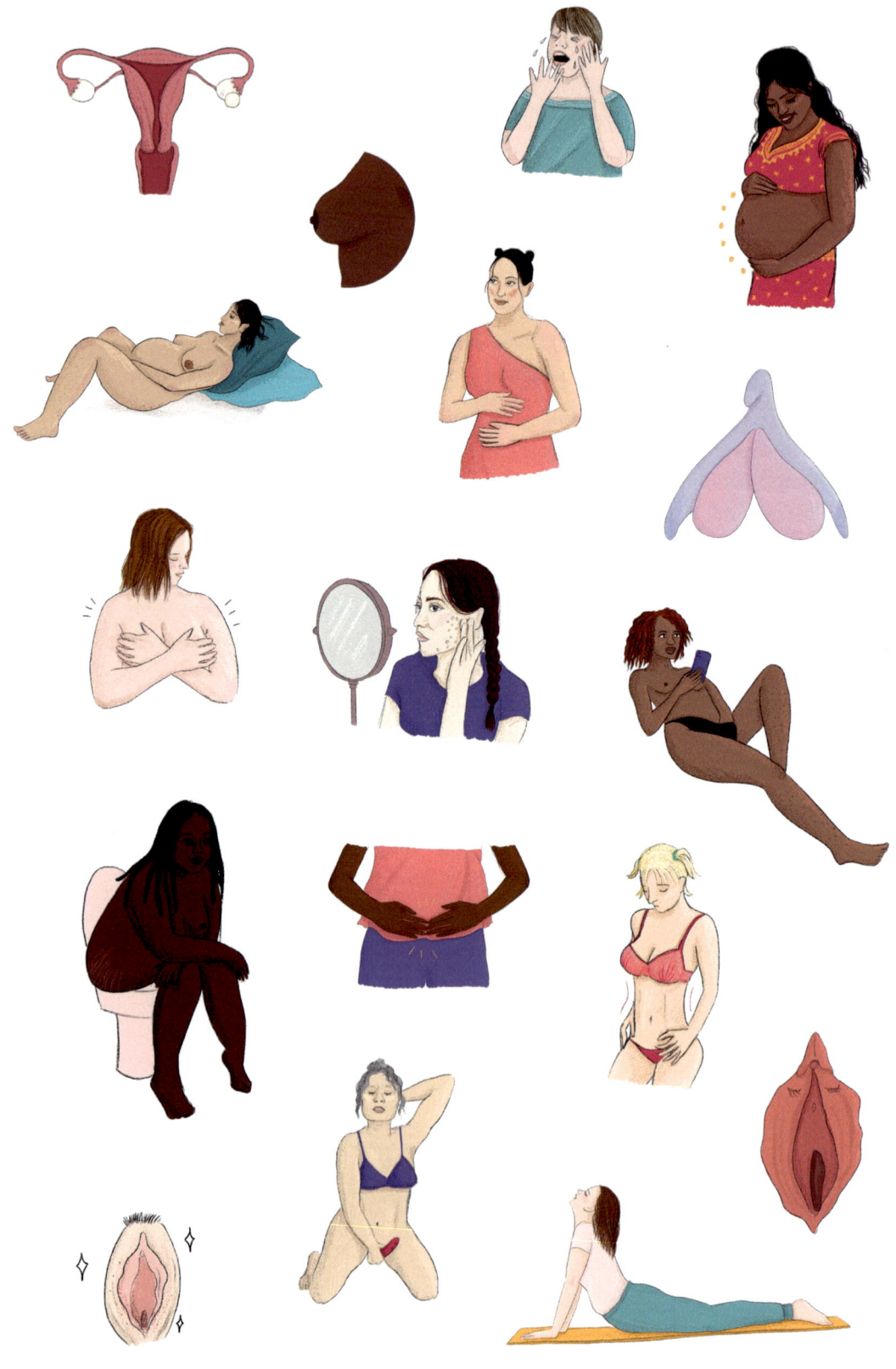

CHAPTER 1

Getting to know your body

Knowing how your reproductive system works is essential for understanding your health at every stage of life. In this chapter, we'll take a comprehensive look at the female anatomy, starting with the external structures and working inward. You'll learn about each organ's structure, function, and its role in maintaining overall health. This knowledge will not only help you to identify what's normal in your own body but will also equip you with the tools to discuss your health confidently and make informed decisions about your care.

Let's start with the anatomy
The vulva

The vulva is the external part of the female genitalia and includes the labia majora, labia minora, clitoris, urethral opening, and vaginal opening. It serves as a protective barrier and plays a central role in sexual arousal, pleasure, and hygiene. Each part of the vulva is unique to the individual and can vary in size, shape, and colour – all of which are completely normal.

Does it really matter if we call it the vagina?

Yes – there is a really common misconception that you can use the term 'vagina' to refer to all of the external female genitalia.

The truth is that although 'vagina' is often used as an umbrella term for everything in the female genitalia, the vagina actually refers to the closed muscular canal that runs from the vulva (the external genitalia, including the labia and clitoris) through to the cervix (the neck of the uterus).

It's really important that we should all be able to name each part of our anatomy correctly; not only does it help to shake off some of the mystery around the area but it can also help you to feel more empowered when speaking about it; whether that's advocating for yourself in a medical setting, sharing your preferences with partners, or just having a chat with friends.

Getting to know the anatomy of your vulva and clitoris through self-exploration is empowering, and very valuable for understanding your body and enhancing your sexual well-being! Self-exploration can also build confidence, which is beneficial when guiding a partner. Knowing what types of touch and stimulation you enjoy enables you to communicate your preferences and boundaries better, creating a more satisfying, intimate experience for both of you.

The clitoris

Next, let's talk about another widely misunderstood part of the anatomy: the clitoris. The clitoris is a highly sensitive organ whose sole function is for pleasure, unlike every other organ in the body, which are actively involved in a bodily function.

It has been so misunderstood that, in fact, a 1486 guide for finding witches, *The Malleus Maleficarum*, suggested the clitoris was the 'devil's teat'.[1] This guide claimed that if there was a protruding nub of tissue between the labia on a woman it would prove her status as a witch. The belief that the clitoris was the source of evil and harm continued into the 1800s, where women who were seen as suffering from 'hysteria' (or even other conditions like cataplexy or epilepsy) were sometimes subject to removal of their clitoris (clitoridectomies).

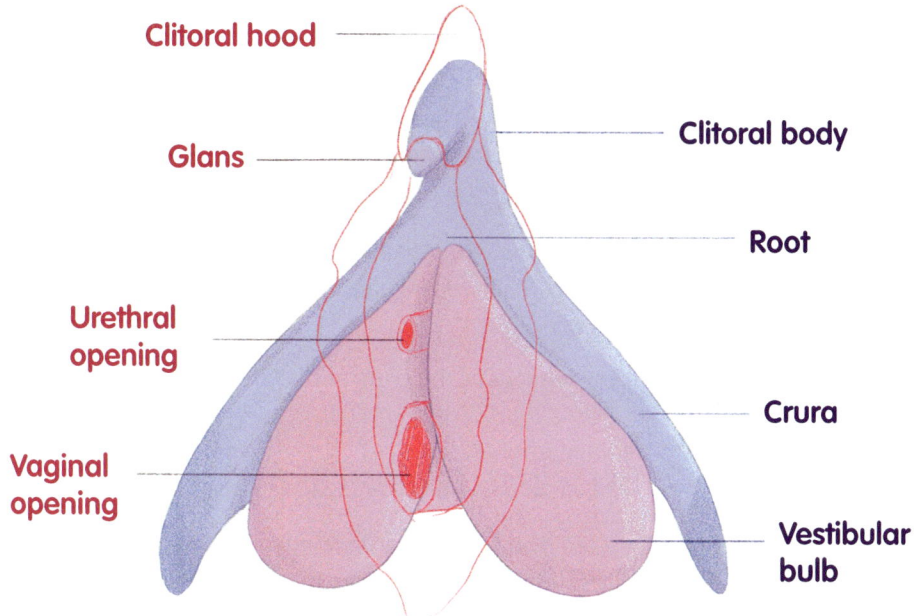

Clitoral hood

Glans

Urethral opening

Vaginal opening

Clitoral body

Root

Crura

Vestibular bulb

Surprisingly it wasn't until 1981 that the Federation of Feminist Women's Health Clinics created anatomically correct images of the clitoris. In 1998, Australian urologist Dr Helen O'Connell published groundbreaking work that revealed the true size and internal structure of the clitoris, showing it to be a much more complex and extensive organ than previously thought.[2] This research has led to a greater understanding of female sexual anatomy.

Where and what is it?

The visible part of the clitoris is situated at the top of the vulva, just above two separate openings: the urethral opening (where urine comes out) and the opening to the vagina.

The actual clitoris consists of several parts; the external parts known as the glans (the visible, bulbous part at the top) and the clitoral hood (a protective flap of skin covering the glans). Deeper beneath the skin surface, the clitoris is shaped like an upside-down wishbone, with a clitoral body branching out to form a V shape. These internal parts extend under the surface of the vulva and can be quite sensitive to stimulation:

- **Body (corpora):** The body of your clitoris is located behind your glans. Think of it as the top of the wishbone that isn't divided. The body extends downward and branches off to form a pair of legs, the crura

- **Crura:** The crura are two legs that extend from the clitoral body. They are the longest part of your clitoris. Together, they form the 'V' of the wishbone and surround your vaginal canal and urethra

- **Vestibular (clitoral) bulbs:** The vestibular bulbs are in-between your crura and your vaginal wall. When feeling aroused, they swell with blood and can even double in size

- **Root:** The root is where the legs of the crura and all the nerves from the erectile tissue meet

What does the clitoris do?

Stimulation of the clitoris can lead to sexual arousal, increased blood flow to the pelvic area, and orgasm. It's important to note that the size and sensitivity of the clitoris can vary from person to person. What works for one person in terms of stimulation may not be the same for another, so communication and exploration with a partner can be essential for sexual satisfaction.

Unlike the male penis, which serves both reproductive and sexual functions, the clitoris does not have a direct role in reproduction. Instead, it exists primarily for sexual pleasure and enjoyment.

The vagina

The vagina is a muscular, elastic canal that connects the vulva to the cervix. It serves multiple purposes: as a passage for menstrual flow, a channel for childbirth, and it is also the typical location for penetrative sexual intercourse. It has its own optimal pH balance and a self-cleaning mechanism that supports healthy bacteria, keeping infections at bay.

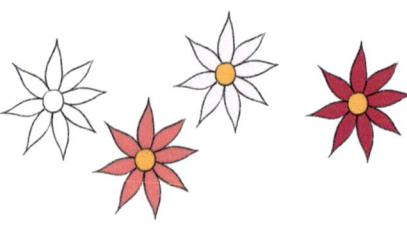

The cervix

Located at the lower end of the uterus, the cervix acts as a gateway between the vagina and the uterus. During your menstruating years, it has a small opening that can slightly enlarge around the time of your period to allow your period blood to escape. It plays its most important role during child-birth, dilating to allow the baby to pass through. The cervix also produces mucus that changes consistency during the menstrual cycle, facilitating or preventing sperm from entering the uterus.

The uterus

Often referred to as the womb, the uterus is a pear-shaped organ, whose primary function is to nourish a fertilised egg, allowing it to implant and develop into a baby during pregnancy. It has muscular walls which can contract during labour to help deliver the baby.

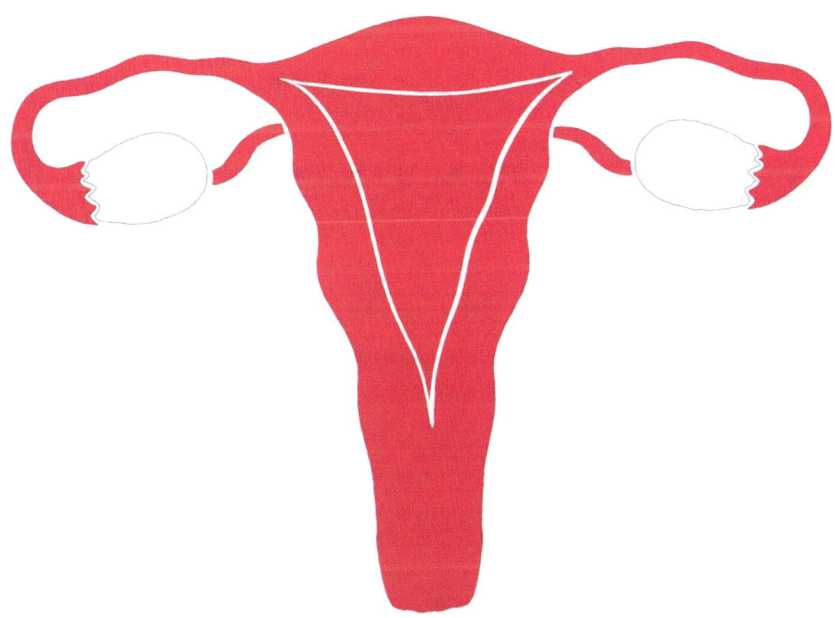

The fallopian tubes

These are narrow tubes that connect the ovaries to the uterus and act as a passage for the egg to move along. Fertilisation typically occurs here, when an egg released from the ovary meets sperm within the tube. The tiny hair-like structures inside the tubes help guide the egg or fertilised embryo towards the uterus. The fallopian tubes are not actually connected directly to the ovaries, but instead they are able to move around and pick up eggs released nearby.

The ovaries

The ovaries are two small, almond-shaped organs located on either side of the uterus. They store your eggs, which develop and mature during each menstrual cycle. One egg is later released from the ovary in the middle of the cycle, a process called ovulation. The ovaries also produce the hormones oestrogen and progesterone, which regulate the menstrual cycle, support pregnancy and help sexual function.

DID YOU KNOW?

The fallopian tube isn't actually connected to the ovary! During ovulation, the ovary releases an egg into the pelvic cavity, and the finger-like fimbriae at the end of the fallopian tube sweep the egg into the tube for its journey towards the uterus. Importantly, the fallopian tubes can move around and even pick up eggs released from either ovary. If one tube is removed, for example, after an ectopic pregnancy, the remaining tube can compensate, increasing its activity to capture eggs from both ovaries.

A NOTE ON FGM

Female genital mutilation (FGM), also known as female circumcision or female genital cutting, involves the partial or complete removal of external female genitalia for non-medical reasons. FGM is often performed for various cultural, social, and religious reasons, although it has no medical benefits and is considered harmful. It is widely considered a violation of human rights, as it can lead to severe physical and psychological consequences.

There are several types of FGM, ranging from less invasive procedures to more extreme forms:

- **Type 1 – Clitoridectomy:** This involves cutting or removal of part, or all, of the clitoris

- **Type 2 – Excision:** In this procedure, both the clitoris and the labia minora (inner lips) are partially or completely removed

- **Type 3 – Infibulation:** This is the most extreme form of FGM. It involves the removal of the clitoris, labia minora, and labia majora (outer lips), followed by the stitching of the remaining tissue, leaving a small opening for urine and menstruation. This opening can be extremely narrow and may require a procedure to release it in order to allow for sexual intercourse or childbirth

- **Type 4 –** Any other forms of trauma to the vulva not otherwise classified: this may include pricking, piercing, incising, scraping, or cutting

The consequences of FGM can be severe and include medical complications such as damage to the urinary tract, as well as mental health implications due to anxiety, post-traumatic stress disorder, and more. In many countries, performing FGM is illegal, and in certain countries it is also illegal to assist anyone travelling to another country to undergo FGM.

CLEANING YOUR VULVA GUIDE

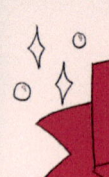

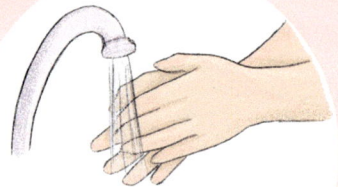

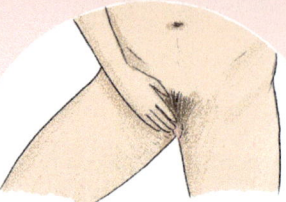

Wash your hands: Begin by thoroughly washing your hands with soap and warm water, this helps prevent the transfer of any harmful bacteria.

Rinse with water: Stand or sit comfortably in the shower or at the sink. Use warm (not hot) water to wet the area around the vulva. This helps loosen debris or discharge.

Apply a small amount of soap to your hand or washcloth and gently cleanse the area, focusing only on the hair-bearing parts. Be sure to avoid getting soap inside the vagina, as this can disrupt the natural pH balance.

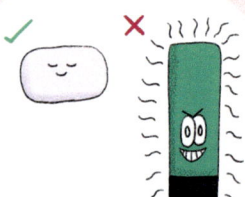

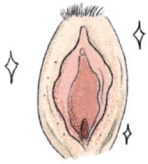

Gentle cleansing (optional): If you choose to use soap, select a mild, fragrance-free and hypo-allergenic option.

Rinse thoroughly: Use clean, warm water to rinse away any soap residue. Ensure that all soap is completely removed from the vulva.

Pat dry, don't rub: Gently pat dry with a clean towel. Avoid vigorous rubbing, as this can cause irritation.

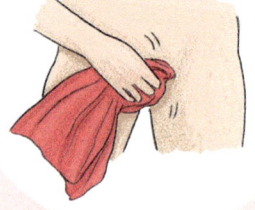

Avoid douching: Douching is not recommended as it can disrupt the natural balance of bacteria in the vagina, leading to irritation or infection.

Front to back: When wiping or cleansing, always move from front to back to prevent the spread of bacteria from the rectal area to the vulva.

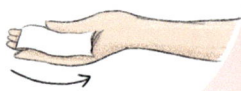

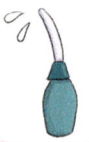

Regular check-ups: Keep up with routine gynaecological exams to ensure overall vaginal health, such as cervical screening.

Wear breathable underwear: Opt for cotton underwear, which allows for better airflow and helps prevent moisture build-up.

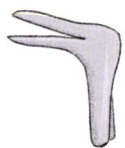

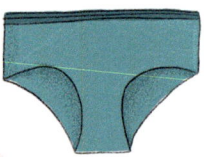

How to clean your genitalia safely

Before we get into how to clean the vulva, it is important to differentiate it from the vagina. Generally, we describe the vagina as 'self-cleaning'.

The vagina is a self-cleaning organ due to its natural, complex ecosystem. Discharge produced by glands within the cervix and vagina is a natural mechanism for cleaning. It helps to remove dead cells, bacteria, and other waste materials. During menstruation, the shedding of the uterine lining helps to remove bacteria and old cells. This process is a natural form of cleansing.

As well as this, the vagina can look after itself because it maintains an acidic pH level (around 3.8 to 4.5), which is inhospitable to many harmful bacteria. This acidity helps to prevent the overgrowth of potentially harmful micro-organisms. The vagina is also home to a community of beneficial bacteria, primarily lactobacilli. These bacteria produce lactic acid, which helps to maintain the acidic pH and create a protective barrier, preventing harmful bacteria from flourishing. Working alongside this,, the vagina has its own immune system, with cells that identify and neutralise harmful pathogens that may enter. Glands in the cervix produce mucus that varies in consistency throughout the menstrual cycle. This mucus helps to trap and flush out foreign particles, dead cells, and pathogens.

All of this means that it is important never to wash inside the vagina (aka douching) or using harsh soaps, which can disrupt this natural balance and lead to infections or irritation.

Therefore, in most cases, it's recommended to allow the vagina to self-clean without intervention. If you're experiencing unusual symptoms, smells or discomfort it is unlikely to be a cleaning issue and it's best to consult a healthcare professional for advice.

However, the hair-bearing parts on the outside, aka the vulva, be cleaned safely.

What happens during the menstrual cycle?

The menstrual cycle is not just another way of talking about your period. In fact, it describes the set of processes and changes that occurs on a repeating basis in women, and individuals with ovaries and a uterus. This series of hormonal and physiological changes occurs in order to prepare the body for the possibility of pregnancy.

While we typically describe the menstrual cycle as lasting around 28 days, it can vary from person to person and also cycle to cycle.

It consists of phases, including menstruation (the shedding of the uterine lining), the follicular phase (preparation of an egg for potential fertilisation), ovulation (the release of a mature egg from the ovary), and the luteal phase (preparation of the uterus for potential implantation of a fertilised egg). If pregnancy does not occur, the cycle restarts, counting the first day of the cycle as the first day of bleeding.

DID YOU KNOW?

If you are on hormonal medications like the combined contraceptive pill, which give you a monthly bleed when you have a break in the medication, this bleed is not technically called menstruation or a period. The correct scientific term is to call it a withdrawal bleed, because it is not a spontaneous bleed but occurs in response to taking a break from the hormones contained in the medication.

Let's understand each phase in a bit more detail

You can think of the menstrual cycle like a house that gets ready for a guest (a potential baby). The house has different rooms, and each room does something special to prepare for the guest.

Here's how it works:

Days 1–5: Menstruation (your period)

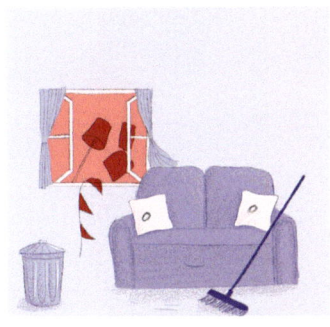

This is like the house getting a little cleaning done and having a clear-out to freshen up for the possibility of guests coming round soon. The old furniture and dust (unused lining from the uterus) is cleaned out and sent away.

The uterine lining, called the endometrium, reaches its thinnest during this phase. The actual duration of bleeding during the period can vary, and a typical period may last up to 8 days, but on average lasts about 5 or 6.

Check out Chapter 2 on periods for more of a deep dive into what is typical, and when to get checked out!

Hormones: Levels of oestrogen and progesterone are typically at their lowest during this part of the cycle. As a result, during the week of your period, you might feel tired, low in motivation, and more emotional. The drop in progesterone hormone is what causes the top layers of the lining to become broken down and leave the body.

Days 6–14: Follicular and proliferative phase

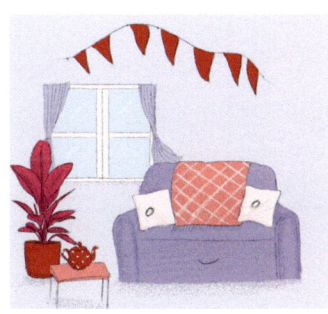

Back to our analogy of the house, in the next phase the house starts to decorate and get all cozy. It's like adding comfy pillows, blankets, and setting the table before the guests arrive.

Within the uterus, the endometrium is thickening up. This is known as proliferation.

The phases of the menstrual cycle

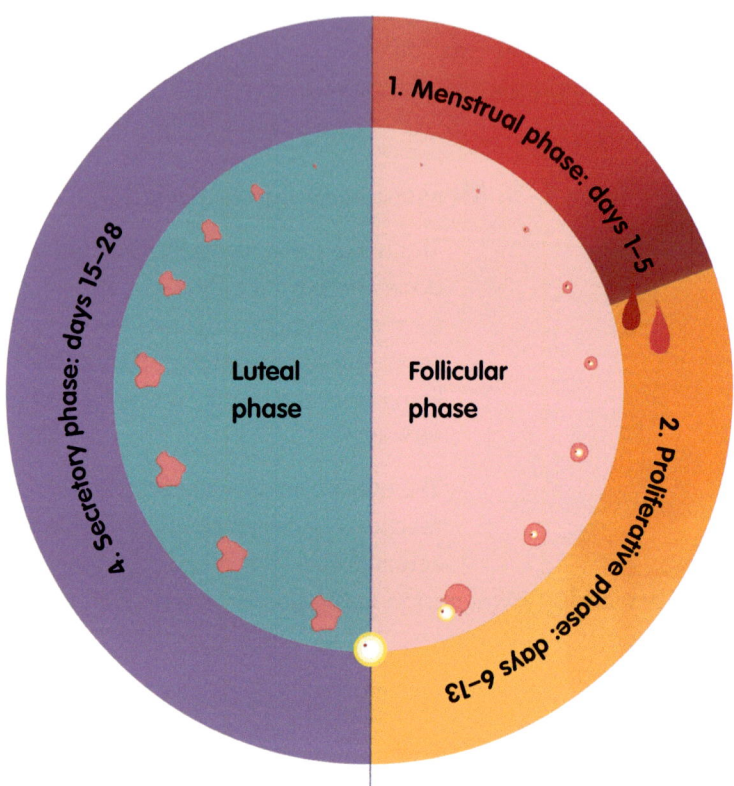

1. Menstrual phase: days 1–5

2. Proliferative phase: days 6–13

3. Ovulation: day 14

4. Secretory phase: days 15–28

Luteal phase

Follicular phase

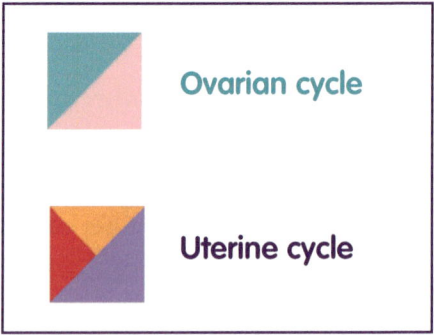

Ovarian cycle

Uterine cycle

Meanwhile, as soon as menstruation begins, the ovaries prepare eggs for release (oocytes). This is known as the follicular phase because multiple follicles develop, and eventually one follicle in one of the ovaries becomes the largest of all the follicles. It is called the dominant follicle and is about the size of a grain of sand (1–2 cm or 0.4–0.8 in).

This follicle is the one preparing to be released at ovulation. For most people, the follicular phase lasts 10–22 days, but this can vary from cycle to cycle.

Hormones: Oestrogen typically rises during this phase. This signals to the uterine lining to grow. The pituitary gland (a small area at the base of the brain that makes hormones) produces a hormone called follicle-stimulating hormone (FSH). FSH tells the ovaries to prepare an egg for ovulation (release of an egg from the ovary). The dominant follicle produces oestrogen as it grows, so your maximum oestrogen levels occur just before ovulation happens.

During the follicular phase, you might feel more energetic, focused, power-ful, and positive thanks to the rising oestrogen levels.

Day 14: Ovulation

This is when the house sends out an invita-tion to the guest (the sperm). It's like putting up a sign that says 'Welcome, come on in!'

The dominant follicle reaches about 2 cm (0.8 in). When it bursts, an egg leaves the ovary and enters the fallopian tube. The release of an egg from an ovary is called ovulation. This egg is ready to be fertilised.

The process of ovulation occurs about midway through the menstrual cycle, but if your cycle is not exactly 28 days long it can be difficult to predict when it will occur. The best way is actually to count 14 days back from your last period. This tells you which day you ovulated on last month. This is because the length of the luteal phase is generally fixed, so around 14 days after you ovulate is when your period will begin. For example, if your cycle is 30 days long, you likely ovulated on day 16.

Sometimes ovulation may not happen at all (anovulation). Anovulation is more common during the first years of having a period, and also during the run-up to menopause, when your ovaries don't have as many eggs available. It can also happen while breastfeeding or with certain conditions, such as polycystic ovarian syndrome (PCOS). When there is no ovulation, the next steps in the cycle may be affected, which can result in irregular or absent periods. (More on PCOS in Chapter 4 on hormones.)

Hormones: The dominant follicle in the ovary produces more and more oestrogen as it grows larger. When oestrogen levels are high enough, they send a signal to the brain. The pituitary gland in the brain then causes a dramatic increase in luteinising hormone (LH). This spike is what causes the release of the egg to occur. Oestrogen levels begin to drop again after ovulation.

At ovulation, you might feel your most confident, sociable, and sexually energised due to peak oestrogen levels and a surge in progesterone. However, some people can actually be aware of ovulation taking place, as they may experience mild pain or cramping, known as mittelschmerz, as the ovary releases an egg.

Days 15–28: Secretory and luteal phase

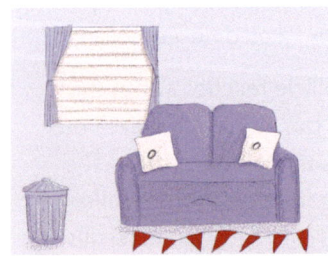

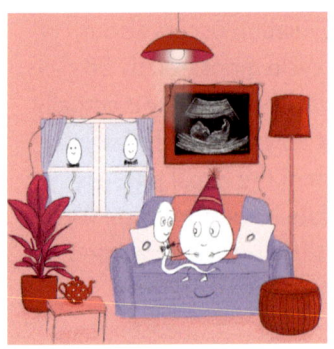

The house now awaits the arrival of its guest. If the guest (the egg) doesn't meet someone (sperm) to dance with, the house will gradually start to take down the decorations and clean up a bit. It's like realising the guest isn't coming this time, so it's time to tidy up and get ready for the next chance.

If the egg does meet sperm, then the house gets really busy preparing for the guest to stay longer!

During this time the lining of the womb (endometrium) continues to develop and mature. If pregnancy doesn't occur, this lining gets broken down again. The cells of the lining make and release many types of chemicals to prepare the endometrium for implantation of the fertilised egg, which is why it is known as the secretory phase.

Hormones: After ovulation, the follicle that held the egg turns into a new organ called a corpus luteum (hence the term 'luteal phase'). It makes the hormones progesterone and oestrogen to support a potential pregnancy until the placenta can take over. If pregnancy does not happen, the corpus luteum breaks down between 9 and 11 days after ovulation. During this phase the progesterone level rises. This causes the uterine lining to stop thickening and start maturing to prepare for a fertilised egg.

If no pregnancy happens, progesterone will peak and then drop. Blood vessels shrink and the uterine lining breaks down. Chemical messengers known as prostaglandins cause the uterine muscle to cramp, which helps to start the period. The uterine cells produce less of these chemicals if pregnancy happens. These hormonal changes can contribute to common premenstrual symptoms. Common symptoms are mood changes, headaches, acne, bloating, and breast tenderness.

A drop in progesterone and oestrogen then triggers your period, and the cycle begins all over again.

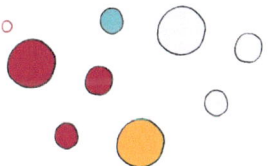

So, there we have it. The menstrual cycle is closely timed to get everything ready for the possibility of having a baby. But, even if pregnancy doesn't occur, it's an important process for keeping the body healthy and ready for the next opportunity.

Remember that hormonal medications do interfere with the natural rise and fall of these hormones, instead keeping the hormone levels constant. This isn't a bad thing as that is why we use these medications in the first place! (More on these medications in Chapter 6 on contraception.)

Reading your discharge

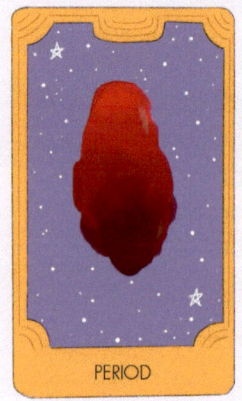

PERIOD

Follicular phase part 1

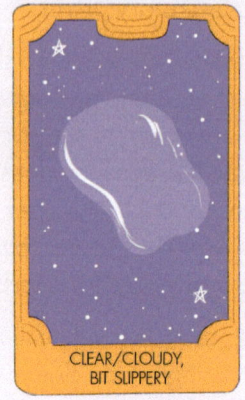

CLEAR/CLOUDY, BIT SLIPPERY

Follicular phase part 2

GLOOPY+ STRETCHY, RESEMBLING EGG WHITES

Pre-ovulation phase

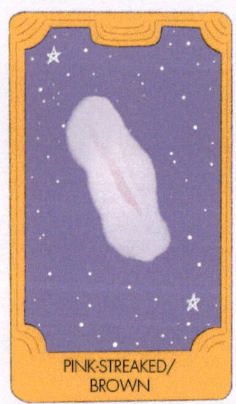

PINK-STREAKED/ BROWN

Ovulation phase

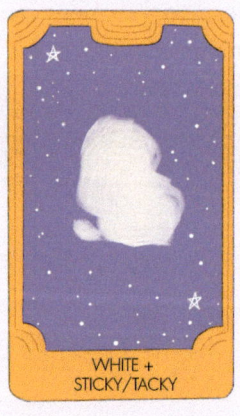

WHITE + STICKY/TACKY

Luteal phase

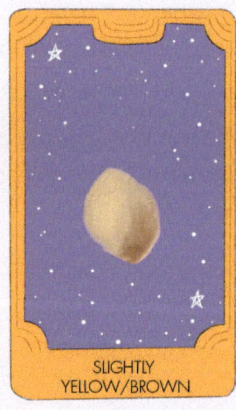

SLIGHTLY YELLOW/BROWN

Premenstrual phase

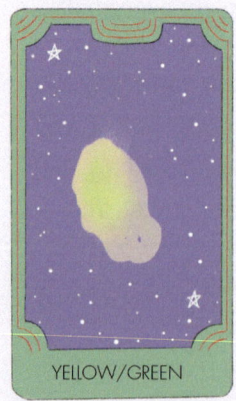

YELLOW/GREEN

Infections such as STIs

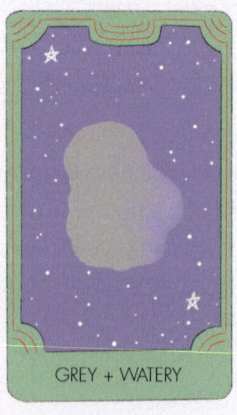

GREY + WATERY

Other infections

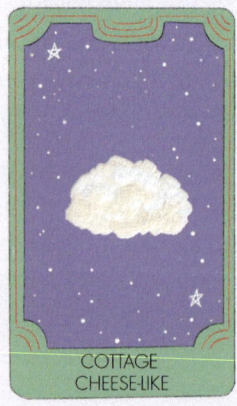

COTTAGE CHEESE-LIKE

Yeast Infection, aka thrush

What actually IS discharge and what does it mean?

From the time you go through puberty and start getting your period, you'll probably notice vaginal discharge in your underwear. This slippery liquid is made of fluids from the cervix, uterus, and vagina, and has several purposes:

1. It is protective – organisms and chemicals in the fluid help keep infections away

2. It reduces the friction from sex to make it more comfortable

3. It can actually help sperm reach the egg during conception!

Depending on the stage of your cycle, you may notice the colour, consistency, volume, and even smell of the discharge can change.

The changing levels of oestrogen throughout the menstrual cycle leads to changes in your cervical discharge, which can provide valuable clues if you are trying to work out where you are in your cycle.

What should it look like during the follicular and ovulation phases?

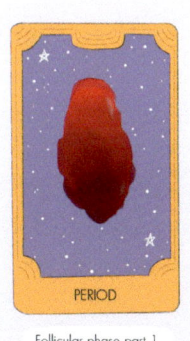

PERIOD

Follicular phase part 1

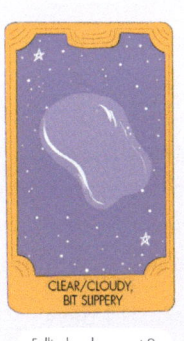

CLEAR/CLOUDY, BIT SLIPPERY

Follicular phase part 2

The early part of the menstrual cycle is the build-up to ovulation, aka the follicular phase.

The first week is your period, but once that clears in the second week you may see around 3–5 days of clear or cloudy discharge that feels a bit slippery.

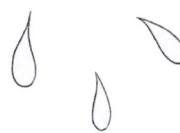

25

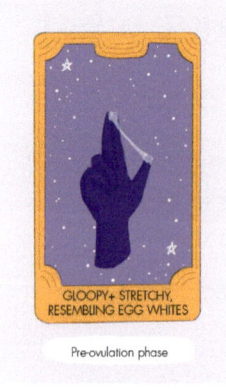

GLOOPY+ STRETCHY, RESEMBLING EGG WHITES

Pre-ovulation phase

As you approach ovulation (towards the end of week 2), the discharge may begin to become more gloopy and stretchy, looking like egg whites. During this time, you could get up to 30 times your usual amount of daily discharge! This type of slippery discharge appears specifically at this point in your cycle, just before ovulation, in order to help support the efforts of any sperm trying to make it to the egg.

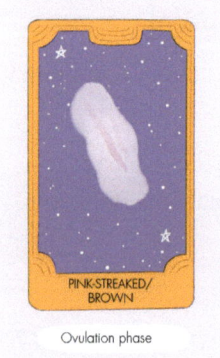

PINK-STREAKED/ BROWN

Ovulation phase

During ovulation itself (around day 14 of the cycle), some people notice a very small amount of bleeding, which may appear as a pink-streaked discharge or a small amount of brown staining in your underwear. While bleeding outside of your period should always be investigated, if it always accompanies ovulation, it may not be something to worry about.

What about in the luteal phase?

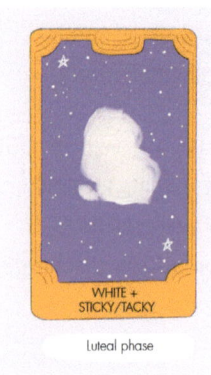

WHITE + STICKY/TACKY

Luteal phase

After ovulation, in the luteal phase (weeks 3 and 4), progesterone levels rise to support the thickened lining of the womb. During this time, you may notice your discharge returning to a white-ish colour. The volume of discharge tends to decrease from here on, and becomes thicker in consistency and possibly even sticky or tacky (like glue).

This can last up to 14 days.

What colour can discharge be during the premenstrual phase/period?

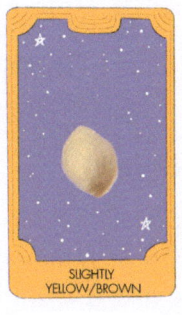

SLIGHTLY
YELLOW/BROWN

Premenstrual phase

Right before your period begins, you may notice mucus that has a yellow or brown colour. This is because when blood moves slowly from the womb to the vagina (aka when the flow is slowly starting), it clots and oxidises on the way out so it looks darker. It can also mix with cervical discharge, giving the yellow appearance.

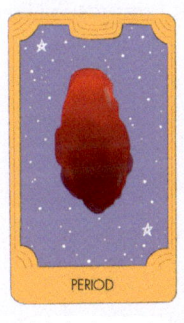

PERIOD

Follicular phase part 1

Period blood can range between bright red and dark brown-black depending on how heavy the flow is and how quickly the blood moves. As your period slows again, you might see some more brown discharge. All of these different shades of red, brown, and black are very normal for a period, and vary significantly from person to person!

Should there be discharge if I'm pregnant?

It's very typical to notice more vaginal discharge during pregnancy, which is usually clear or white in colour. The body produces this increased discharge for a reason; to reduce the risk of any infections travelling from the vagina up to the uterus where the fetus is developing. As you progress in your pregnancy, you may see the amount of discharge increase due to rising oestrogen hormone levels.

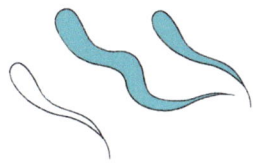

What about the other colours?

It is important to note any changes in your vaginal discharge – you should already be familiar with what is normal for you so you can recognise when it changes! For example, when you track your periods, you can also track your discharge throughout the month and the different colours that you see on different days.

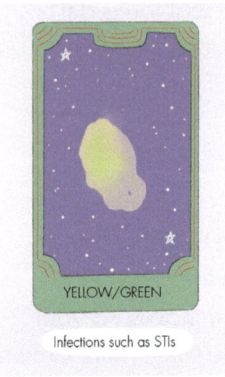

YELLOW/GREEN

Infections such as STIs

Yellow or green discharge

A yellow or greenish discharge, especially if frothy or accompanied by an unpleasant odour, may indicate a sexually-transmitted infection like chlamydia or trichomoniasis. A doctor or nurse can take a quick swab and let you know if any antibiotics are needed. (More about sexually transmitted infections (STIs) in the sex chapter!)

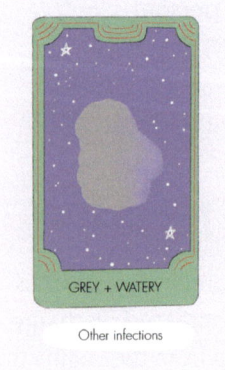

GREY + WATERY

Other infections

Grey discharge

Grey watery vaginal discharge may also be a sign of an infection like bacterial vaginosis (BV). If you notice grey discharge along with itching, irritation, a strong smell or redness around the vagina, you should visit your doctor to start the appropriate treatment.

White discharge

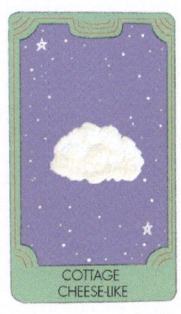

COTTAGE
CHEESE-LIKE

Yeast Infection, aka thrush

A thick, white discharge resembling cottage cheese, often accompanied by itching, discomfort, or soreness, may suggest a yeast infection, commonly known as thrush. While this condition is generally treatable with over-the-counter antifungal medications, if you get these symptoms frequently make sure you get properly checked to ensure your symptoms are definitely due to thrush, and that the infection is not resistant to the over-the-counter treatments.

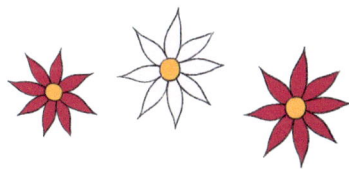

So, there you have it; now you are equipped to understand the different rainbow of colours of discharge you might see during your cycle. White, clear, pink, red, brown, and even black can all be expected at different times in the month. Yellow, green, or grey should be checked out so you don't miss any infections that need treating.

Now that we have explored the key anatomical landmarks of the female reproductive system and taken a closer look at what happens throughout the menstrual cycle, we have a great foundational understanding of how your body works. By understanding the anatomy and physiology behind these systems, you can get to know what is normal for you and when to get checked out.

Top tips for relieving period cramps

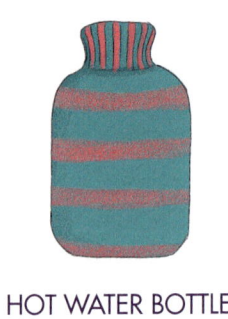

HOT WATER BOTTLE

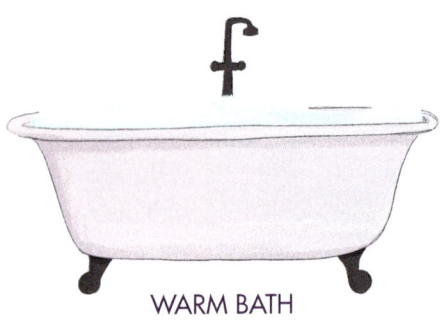

WARM BATH

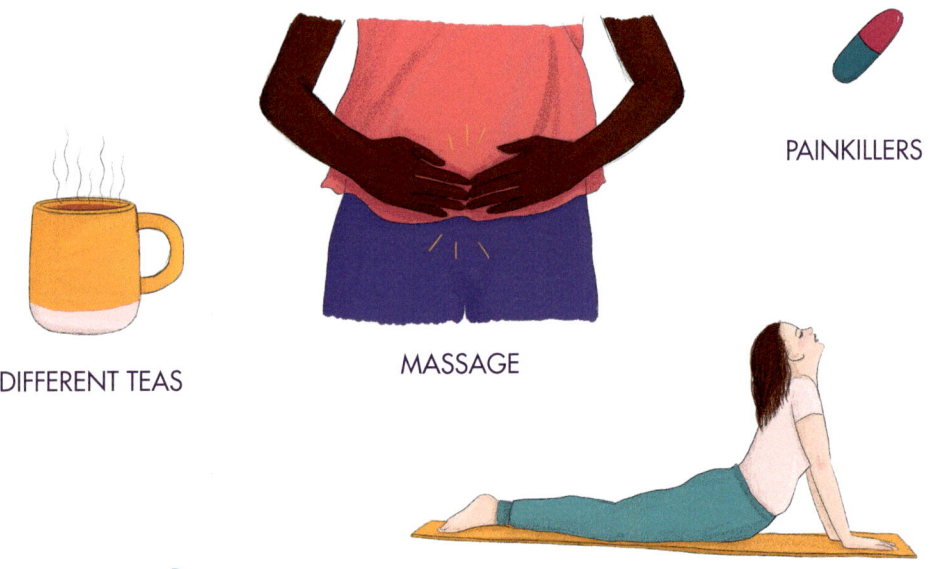

DIFFERENT TEAS

MASSAGE

PAINKILLERS

GENTLE EXERCISE

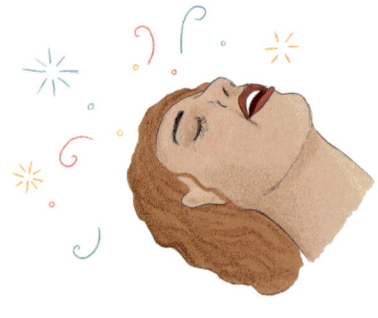

ORGASM

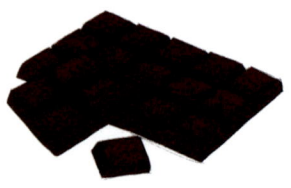

DARK CHOCOLATE

CHAPTER 2

Periods

From the very beginning of puberty, it becomes apparent to most of us that it is impossible to compare periods; every person who experiences them has their own unique journey. While exactly what we experience throughout our menstrual cycles will be personal to us all, there are some common themes, and knowing what is 'normal', or typical, can help us to work out if our own periods are something we should be concerned about.

What is a period?

Your menstrual period is specifically defined as the shedding of the uterine lining, resulting in vaginal bleeding, which occurs in response to a drop in progesterone hormone levels. Technically, the day the bleeding begins becomes the first day of your menstrual cycle.

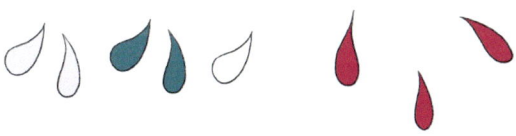

DID YOU KNOW?

Period blood is not the same as the blood flowing through your veins!

It's a combination of blood, old uterine tissue, vaginal mucous lining cells, and bacteria from the vaginal flora. These secretions include water, electrolytes, proteins, and enzymes, and the fluid contains less iron and other blood components than typical blood.

One major difference is that menstrual blood doesn't clot like regular blood from a cut. It contains fewer platelets and clotting factors, which prevents it from forming scabs, allowing it to flow freely during your period.

What is 'normal' for periods?

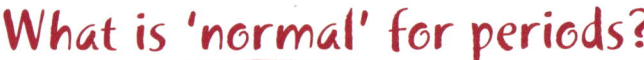

- Your cycle lies within the range 24–38 days
- Periods last less than 8 days
- Cycle length should be roughly similar each month, varying by no more than 20 days between the shortest and longest cycle
- They don't interfere with your ability to do your usual activities. This means they are not too heavy or too painful, so you are still able to go to school or work even on the heaviest days

How often should they come?

An average menstrual cycle lasts 28 days, although it is normal for the length of your cycle to vary by a few days more or less each month. This variation can be even more noticeable if you are still going through puberty, as it can take several years for ovulation to become regular and for the cycles to become more predictable.

One of the most empowering things you can do for your menstrual health is to track your cycle day by day; you can do this using good old-fashioned pen and paper, or download one of the many period-tracking apps now available for your phone. You input the dates of your period and what happens, so you can calculate the length of your cycles and check in the box on page 32 to see whether it falls within the normal level of variation.

DID YOU KNOW?

While many people feel like their entire cycle varies month to month, it is actually only the first half of your cycle that can vary in length as the second half is fixed. This all relates to when ovulation takes place. Ovulation is the release of a mature egg from one of the ovaries, typically occurring midway through the menstrual cycle, making it the most fertile time for conception. Once you have ovulated, you will usually see a period around 14 days later. However, anything that affects whether you ovulate on time can mean the first half of the cycle can be shorter or longer. (More on this in Chapter 4 on hormones!)

This information is particularly useful if you are trying to conceive with irregular cycles. If you are trying to predict when you will ovulate, you need to count backwards from your last period to work out when it will happen. In a 24-day cycle, you actually ovulated on day 10!

Which is the best choice of period product for me?

There are several different types of period products available, each with its own features and benefits. The choice of a period product depends on individual preferences, comfort, lifestyle, flow intensity, and environmental concerns.

Here are some common period products and reasons why someone might choose each one:

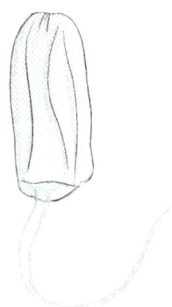

1 Tampons:

- **Pros:** Tampons are discreet and can be worn during most activities, including swimming. They are inserted into the vagina and absorb blood before it leaves the body

- **Considerations:** Some people may find tampons uncomfortable, and there's a rare risk of toxic shock syndrome if not changed regularly. As they need to be inserted into the vagina, they can be uncomfortable or take some time to get used to if someone has never been sexually active before

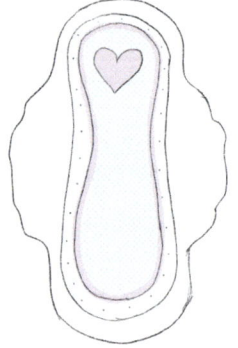

2 Period pads (available as disposable and reusable):

- **Pros:** Pads are easy to use and don't require insertion. They come in various sizes and absorbencies, making them suitable for different flow levels. Reusable cloth pads are an eco-friendly option

- **Considerations:** Pads can sometimes feel bulky, and there's a potential for leaks if not changed regularly. They are often not that discreet to

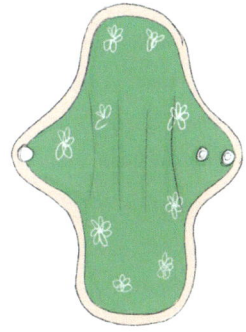

change, with noisy rustles of the wrappers, and they can often move about on your underwear if the adhesive doesn't stick properly

The majority of the disposable period pads do contain plastic, so they are not recyclable, but many of the manufacturers are gradually offering more plastic-free options

3 Menstrual cups:

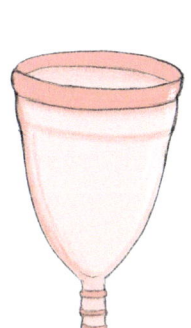

- **Pros:** Cups are inserted into the vagina to collect menstrual blood, then they are removed, emptied, rinsed, and reinserted again. Menstrual cups are eco-friendly and cost-effective as they hold more fluid than most tampons or pads. This also makes them suitable for heavy flows and can allow for longer wear – up to 12 hours in some cases – so they can be particularly convenient for busy lifestyles or overnight use. Many people find cups more comfortable, as they do not cause dryness and are made from medical-grade silicone, which is hypoallergenic

  Environmentally, a cup is a sustainable choice, generating significantly less waste than traditional menstrual products. A single cup can last up to 10 years with proper care. Additionally, they can help users better understand their menstrual flow and anatomy, fostering greater body awareness

- **Considerations:** Menstrual cups can sometimes cause discomfort or irritation, particularly if not inserted correctly or if the fit isn't ideal for the user's anatomy. Additionally, they require careful cleaning, and the insertion/removal process can feel challenging (and sometimes a bit messy), especially for beginners, as there is a learning curve while you get the hang of the process

4   Menstrual discs:

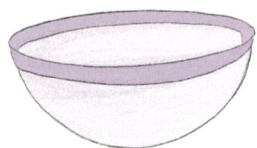

- **Pros:** Menstrual discs are similar to cups but are positioned higher in the vagina and can hold a significant amount of fluid. They may be suitable for people with a heavy flow or those looking for mess-free period sex

- **Considerations:** Like cups, there can be a learning curve for insertion and removal

5. Menstrual underwear:

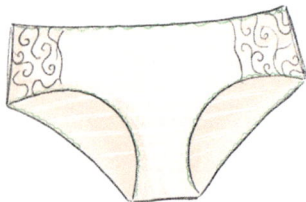

- **Pros:** Menstrual underwear (aka period pants) are convenient and eco-friendly. They can be worn alone or as backup with other products. They offer good protection against leaks and are easy to wash with your usual laundry. They are often a perfect choice for teenagers just getting comfortable with periods who are looking for a discreet option to use at school

- **Considerations:** Some people may not find them suitable for very heavy flows, as they may need to change the underwear multiple times during the day. They need to be washed between uses so the user needs to have a few pairs in supply

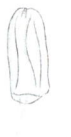 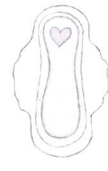 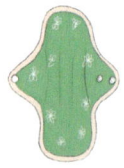 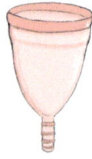 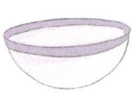 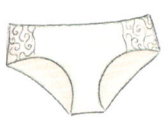

Ultimately, the choice of a period product is a personal decision. It's important to consider factors like comfort, absorbency needs, lifestyle, environmental concerns, and any medical conditions you may have. Trying different products to see what works best for you is often the most effective way to find the right fit.

Irregular periods

There are many possible causes of irregular periods, and, if you aren't trying to get pregnant, having unpredictable periods is not necessarily something to be too concerned about. However, if you are not on any hormonal medication, it is important to have a period at least every 3 months. Otherwise, the lining of the womb can continue to get thicker and thicker. This can be risky if left long term as it may develop into something called endometrial hyperplasia.

If your periods are very infrequent it is worth discussing with your doctor to see if there is any cause, and whether anything can be done to make them more regular.

Common causes of irregular periods include:

- **Puberty:** During the first few years after periods begin, it is common to have some anovulatory cycles, meaning that there are some months where no egg is released. This can mean that irregular periods are very common for the first 2 years, but it can take as long as 8 years before your periods settle into a predictable, regular cycle

- **Polycystic ovary syndrome (PCOS) and endometriosis:** These conditions can cause cysts to form on your ovaries, which can interfere with the development of follicles and ovulation

- **Extreme weight loss or weight gain, excessive exercise or stress:** These can affect your brain's production of the hormones involved in the menstrual cycles. Stress can also include any unexpected physical stresses on our bodies, such as if you are doing lots of travel and shifting time zones, or when you have a vaccination; any of these things can disrupt your hormone cycles temporarily and lead to a few months of irregular cycles

- **Thyroid problems:** Changes to the thyroid hormone can disrupt the hormone signals from the brain that trigger ovulation, leading to irregular cycles

- **The perimenopause:** As the supply of eggs in the ovaries begins to run out, anovulatory cycles become more common meaning periods become irregular, either more frequent or more spaced out. (More on this in Chapter 9 on the menopause!)

- **Early pregnancy:** If your period is unusually late, it is always a good idea to take a pregnancy test!
- **Forms of hormonal contraception:** Contraception that contains proges-terone, such as the combined pill or the intrauterine coil, cause the lining of the womb to stay thin, and may cause your periods to stop or your bleeding may instead be very light and infrequent. In this scenario, not having a regular bleed is not necessarily a cause for concern but, instead, it is just part of how the medication is working

Ideally, women should have a minimum four periods per year if they are not on any hormonal medication. If your periods are more irregular than this, your doctor may be able to prescribe medication to stimulate a bleed in order to keep the lining of the womb thin.

Being aware of your monthly pattern is the first step to taking control of your cycles!

True or false?

1. Having a regular bleed is important to be healthy

False! Several cultural misconceptions contribute to the belief that women need to have regular periods even when on hormonal medication. One is the belief that experiencing a monthly period is necessary to mimic the natu-ral menstrual cycle, despite the fact that hormonal contraceptives effectively manage the endometrial lining without the need for a bleed. Additionally, some cultures view menstruation as a form of bodily cleansing or detoxifica-tion, though there is no scientific basis for this belief. The endometrium does not store toxins; it merely prepares for potential pregnancy and therefore there is no biological need for the regular shedding apart from preventing hyperplasia.

2. Not having a monthly bleed can lead to future infertility

False! Although having a monthly period is a good sign that you are ovulating spontaneously, suppressing the monthly period with hormonal contraception does not negatively impact future fertility.

Hormonal contraception does not cause a long-term impact on fertility because its effects are fully reversible once the method is discontinued.

After stopping hormonal contraceptives like the pill, patch, or injection, most people's menstrual cycle and ovulation resume within a few weeks to months, depending on individual factors. While some users may experience a short delay in the return of regular cycles, this is frustrating, but usually temporary, unless the pill has been masking an underlying condition such as PCOS or premature ovarian insufficiency. Historically, early versions of birth control pills were designed to include a withdrawal bleed to reassure women that they were not pregnant, reinforcing the belief that a monthly period is necessary.

Regular menstrual cycles can be a good sign of well-being, but hormonal contraceptives can safely regulate the endometrial lining without the need for withdrawal bleeds, challenging traditional misconceptions about the necessity of monthly periods.

DID YOU KNOW?

Maintaining a thin endometrial lining is crucial for several reasons. Primarily, it reduces the risk of endometrial hyperplasia, a condition where the lining becomes excessively thick and can increase the risk of endometrial cancer due to prolonged exposure to unopposed oestrogen. Additionally, a thin endometrium which is shed regularly helps to prevent abnormal uterine bleeding, which can lead to significant discomfort and health issues, such as anaemia, due to excessive blood loss.

We recommend having a minimum of four menstrual bleeds per year to avoid the build-up of the endometrial lining that can lead to hyperplasia. Regular menstrual cycles also serve as an indicator of overall reproductive health, signalling that hormonal cycles are functioning properly.

However, for women on hormonal contraceptives, regular withdrawal bleeds or periods are not necessary for maintaining health. Hormonal contraceptives regulate and thin the endometrial lining, reducing the risk of endometrial hyperplasia even without regular bleeds. The synthetic hormones in these medications maintain the endometrial lining in a thin, stable state, preventing complications associated with a thickened endometrium.

How heavy is too heavy?

Most women will lose around 30–40 ml of blood during their period although the normal range is 5–80 ml.[2] It can be hard to visualise that amount of blood in reality, but using a menstrual cup can help you to gauge how much blood you are losing. However, what seems heavy for one woman may feel completely normal for another.

Is my period heavy?

Your period is described as heavy if you lose more than 80 ml of blood across the duration of your period, or if your periods last for 7 days or longer.

Your bleeding would also be considered heavy if:

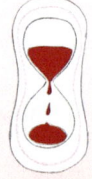

- You have to change your sanitary products every 1–2 hours throughout the day

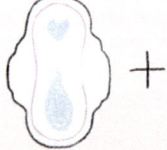

- You sometimes bleed (flood) through to your clothes or bedding when you are asleep at night

- You need to double up on sanitary products (e.g., tampons and pads) to prevent leaks

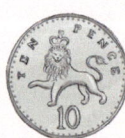

- You need to wake up in the night to change your tampon/ pad or empty your menstrual cup

- You regularly pass blood clots larger than 2.5 cm (about the size of a 10-pence coin)

For about half of women, there is no underlying cause for heavy periods. However, if you think your period is excessively heavy for you, then seeing your own doctor can help decide if further testing would be useful to identify any underlying issue.

Most importantly, if your periods are heavy enough to have an impact on you being able to live your life and leave your house, then this is not something you need to accept and live with forever!

What does 80 ml of blood look like?

By the medical definitions, losing more than 80 ml blood in a week is considered heavy but, as you can imagine, 80 ml is actually not a lot of blood. It can be difficult to tell how much blood you are losing during your period because the appearance can vary depending on the type of period product you're using. If you are expecting 80 ml across 5 days, then you can expect around 15–20 ml per day.

Here's an approximate idea of what it might look like in different period products:

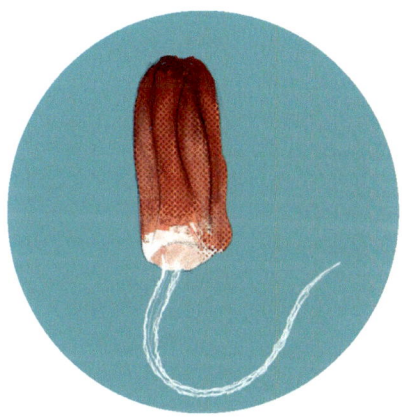

- **Tampons:** Tampons are designed to absorb liquid and expand, so not all the blood can be easily seen. However, if you were to unravel a fully saturated tampon, it might appear as a reddish or brownish discolouration on the tampon material. A fully saturated regular tampon can hold about 5–10 ml of blood, which is roughly equivalent to 1–2 teaspoons

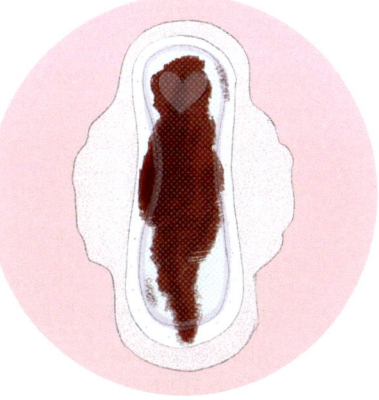

- **Pads:** On a pad, menstrual blood spreads out and covers a significant portion of the pad's surface area, likely creating a noticeable and larger stain. Pads are designed to capture and contain menstrual flow on their absorbent surface. A fully saturated regular sanitary pad can typically hold about 5–10 ml of blood, similar to a regular tampon. This can vary slightly depending on the brand and type of pad

  o Reusable sanitary pads hold a similar amount of blood but have the added benefit of being plastic-free and washable

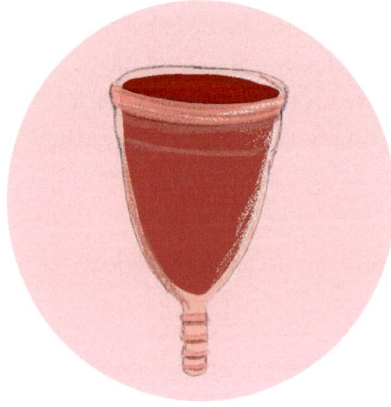

- **Menstrual cups:** Blood in a menstrual cup is much easier to quantify, because it is not absorbed, and the cups usually have some markings on the side so you can see the approximate volume held. A menstrual cup can hold significantly more volume than a regular tampon or pad. Depending on the size and brand, a menstrual cup typically holds a maximum of 20–30 ml of blood, which is about three to six times more than a regular tampon or pad. This makes it a convenient option for longer wear without needing frequent changes

- **Menstrual underwear:** Some menstrual underwear brands have different absorbency levels but most are black in colour, which effectively masks blood stains, making it easier to clean and maintain. The blood in menstrual underwear is distributed throughout the crotch area, creating a noticeable darkened or wet appearance. This makes them very discreet but it is nearly impossible to quantify the amount of blood absorbed!

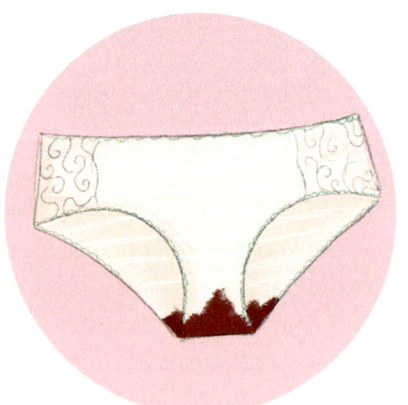

  o Typically, period underwear is designed to hold anywhere from 10 ml to 50 ml of blood, with higher absorbency pairs capable of holding up to the equivalent of four regular tampons

Causes of heavy bleeding

Some conditions of the womb and ovaries can cause heavy bleeding, including:

- **Fibroids:** These are non-cancerous growths or masses that develop in or around the womb. They are very common, 70–80% of women under the age of 50 may have them,[3] and for most people they don't cause any issues. However, depending on their location, size, and number they can lead to heavy periods and discomfort

- **Endometrial polyps:** These are also non-cancerous growths in the lining of the womb or cervix (neck of the womb), which can contribute to heavy bleeding during periods. If identified on an ultrasound or a procedure called a hysteroscopy, they can be easily removed

- **Endometriosis:** Cells similar to the tissue that lines the womb (endometrium) may be found outside the womb, such as in the ovaries and fallopian tubes. The growth of this tissue can lead to inflammation, which may increase the production of hormones called prostaglandins, making periods heavier (and often painful!). More on endometriosis below!

- **Adenomyosis:** Adenomyosis is a condition similar to endometriosis, and can also cause heavy periods because endometrial tissue grows into the muscle of the uterus itself, leading to an enlarged and thickened uterus. This disrupts how the uterus can squeeze (or contract), making it harder to control blood flow, and creates a bigger surface area to shed from, resulting in heavier and prolonged menstrual bleeding

- **Blood clotting disorders, such as Von Willebrand disease:** If your blood doesn't clot properly, it's harder to stop the bleeding during your period. This can cause prolonged and heavier periods because the body struggles to control the blood loss

- **Underactive thyroid gland (hypothyroidism):** If the thyroid gland does not produce enough thyroid hormone it may cause symptoms such as tiredness and weight gain. The lack of thyroid hormone also interferes with signals that lead to ovulation, making periods irregular and allowing the lining of the womb to build up more, leading to heavier and longer periods when they do occur

- **Womb (endometrial) cancer:** Endometrial cancer can lead to heavy bleeding because the cancerous cells in the uterine lining cause abnormal tissue growth and disruption of normal shedding, resulting in excessive or irregular bleeding. This can include heavier periods, bleeding between periods, or post-menopausal bleeding, which differs from normal heavy periods that follow a predictable cycle. It is important to remember that this is very rare in pre-menopausal women, and for most people heavy periods do not mean cancer

An important feature is that in endometrial cancer the change will usually be dramatic, and sudden; your bleeding pattern is noticeably different to how it was before. Additionally, endometrial cancer may present with other symptoms like pelvic pain, unusual discharge, or abdominal fullness, which are not typically associated with normal menstruation. If you are concerned, it's crucial to speak to a health professional who may arrange an ultrasound or biopsy to rule out cancer

Period cramps

Period pains usually feel like cramps in your abdomen, back, or thighs. These cramps occur in response to hormones and substances like prostaglandins, which are released by the lining of the uterus as it prepares to shed. Prosta-glandins help the uterus to contract and relax, so that the endometrium can detach and flow out of your body.

It is common to feel cramps just before or at the time bleeding starts, and they can continue for 1–3 days. While contractions of the uterus, which is what causes the pain, is a normal part of menstruating, if these pains affect your ability to live a normal life, this may not be normal.

Are these 'normal' or typical cramps?

These factors are typically felt with 'normal' period cramps:

- **Timing:** Cramps usually begin 1–2 days before or at the start of menstruation and last 2–3 days
- **Location:** The pain is typically felt in the lower abdomen but can also radiate to the lower back and thighs

- **Severity:** Cramps range from mild discomfort to moderate pain, but should be manageable

- **Impact:** While cramps can be uncomfortable, they should not prevent you from carrying out daily activities like going to school or work

- **Relief:** Pain usually responds well to non-prescription medications (e.g., ibuprofen or paracetamol) or heat therapy, such as a warm bath or heating pad

If the pain is severe, doesn't respond to typical treatments, or significantly interferes with daily life, it could be a sign of a more serious condition like endometriosis. Tracking when the pain occurs and how bad it is can help inform discussions with your doctors and assist them in working out why this pain may be affecting you.

Is there a cause for my painful periods?

The medical term for painful periods is dysmenorrhea. While cramps are often dismissed as just being part and parcel of menstruating, it is actually not normal to have significant pain with your periods.

If you are someone who has painful cramps but there is no underlying cause, we call this 'primary dysmenorrhoea'. We don't know why some people experience more pain than others, but we do often find that painful periods can run in families.

'Secondary dysmenorrhea' means there is an underlying cause for the pain (such as endometriosis or pelvic inflammatory disease (PID)).

There are some features that may suggest there is an underlying cause for the pain, such as:

- Pain that starts after several years of painless periods

- Pain that occurs at other times of the month, but is exacerbated by menstruation

- Other symptoms, including:
  - o Pain with sex
  - o Difficulty falling pregnant
  - o Non-gynaecological symptoms, such as rectal pain and bleeding

Possible underlying causes for painful periods include:

- Endometriosis
- Adenomyosis
- Fibroids
- Pelvic inflammatory disease

Common conditions that might affect your periods

Endometriosis and adenomysosis

Endometriosis is a condition that many people with periods struggle with, and it's much more than just a cause of painful periods. While pain is often the most noticeable symptom, endometriosis can impact many aspects of life, from fertility to emotional well-being. It can make everyday activities harder, with symptoms sometimes affecting work, relationships, and overall quality of life.

Endometriosis is one of the most common gynaecological illnesses, affecting approximately 10% of all women of reproductive age.[4] It can be a difficult condition to diagnose early, because some people don't experience symptoms, and confirming a diagnosis requires surgery, which has its own risks attached. As a result of this, the average delay from first developing symptoms to receiving a diagnosis is 8 years!

What is endometriosis?

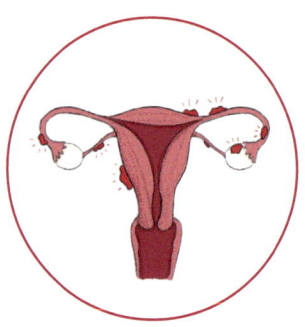

The endometrium is the name for the lining of the womb, which is shed each month at the start of the menstrual cycle. When tissue that is similar to the cells of the endometrium grow outside the womb, such as in the pelvis or on the ovaries, this is known as endometriosis. This tissue can induce a chronic inflammatory reaction that may result in scar tissue formation.

The cells can also bleed in response to the hormones of the menstrual cycle, and this can cause significant pain during your period. The pain can arise in unusual locations such as a specific point in the pelvis or in the rectum depending on where the endometriosis has deposited.

Sometimes these cells form large cysts in the ovaries, known as endometriomas that can also be a source of pain.

What is adenomysosis?

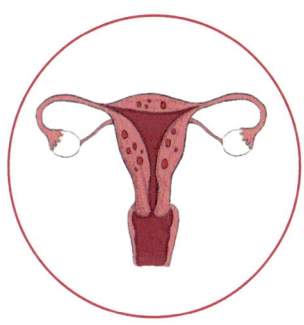

Adenomyosis is a condition that is related to endometriosis, where the endometrial tissue invades into the muscular layer of the uterus. This can make the uterus larger and can cause symptoms like heavy, painful periods, cramping, and discomfort during sex.

The two conditions have similarities and can share symptoms, and some women with endometriosis also have adenomyosis.

What causes endometriosis?

We still don't know exactly why endometriosis happens, but there are a number of theories that put forward various possible causes. It is believed that endometriosis arises when endometrial cells are shed during your period and travel the wrong way (known as retrograde menstruation), travelling through the fallopian tubes and into the pelvis instead of leaving your body as a period. It has also been proposed that there may be a change in your immune system, which means your body doesn't recognise that these endometrium cells shouldn't be there and destroy them.

Some research suggests that your genetics may make you more likely to have endometriosis, because if your mother or sister is affected, you are six times more likely to have endometriosis too![5]

What do the stages mean?

In treating endometriosis, the focus should be primarily on managing symptoms rather than the stage of the disease. This is because the type or severity of endometriosis does not always correlate to the symptoms and individual experiences. This means that two individuals with different stages

47

of endometriosis may experience different symptoms. A woman with mild endometriosis could have severe pain, while someone with more extensive disease might experience little to no discomfort. Therefore, treatment plans should always be personalised.

The stage of endometriosis is usually confirmed by laparoscopy, which is an invasive surgery. However, you don't need to have a laparoscopy to determine the stage of endometriosis before starting treatment. Many doctors can make a diagnosis based on a patient's symptoms, medical history, and non-invasive tests like ultrasound or MRI scans, which can detect signs of endometriosis such as cysts or adhesions.

A laparoscopy, which is ultimately the gold standard for definitive diagnosis, is an invasive procedure and is generally recommended only if symptoms are severe, if there are concerns about fertility, or if other treatments have not been effective. At laparoscopy, doctors can see where endometriosis is deposited and identify other features such as cysts on the ovaries. For some people, endometriosis can cause adhesions, which is scar tissue that sticks the organs together – for example, the uterus and bowel.

To classify the stage of endometriosis, most doctors use a classification system outlined by the American Society for Reproductive Medicine (ASRM).[6] This classifies the condition into four stages based on how much tissue has grown outside the uterus, and how scarring is present.

Stage I (Minimal) involves only a few small patches of tissue with little scarring. Stage II (Mild) has more tissue and some small adhesions. Stage III (Moderate) shows larger lesions, deeper tissue growth, and moderate scarring, often involving the ovaries. Stage IV (Severe) is the most advanced, with widespread tissue growth, large cysts, and significant scarring that can affect other organs by invading into the bladder or bowels. The downside of this system is that it focuses on the physical extent of the disease and doesn't always reflect the severity of symptoms, as some women with lower stages may have worse pain than those with more advanced stages. Not all endometriosis progresses in a stepwise way, going from stage I to IV. Instead, it may remain minimal, or it might progress quickly.

Is endometriosis the same as bad period pain?

Not all painful periods mean endometriosis, and not all endometriosis cause period pain. While many people experience cramps during menstruation, endometriosis also involves other features such as chronic pelvic pain, pain during intercourse, painful bowel movements or urination, and even infertility. These symptoms are usually more severe and persistent than regular period pain. The pain from endometriosis often occurs throughout the month, not just during menstruation, and can be debilitating for many people.

How will I know if I have endometriosis?

The diagnosis of endometriosis is first suspected based on the symptoms you tell your doctor, and then investigated by physical examination and scans such as an ultrasound or MRI scan of your pelvis. Ultimately, the best type of test to confirm a diagnosis of endometriosis is a laparoscopy, which is keyhole surgery to look inside the abdomen and see any endometriosis directly.

However, if your doctor suspects endometriosis, they sometimes recommend starting medical treatment for endometriosis before confirming the diagnosis with laparoscopy. This is because treating the symptoms early can help manage pain and improve quality of life.

Medical treatments, such as hormonal therapies (e.g., contraceptive pills, or hormone blockers such as gonadotropin-releasing hormone (GnRH) agonists), can help reduce inflammation, shrink endometrial tissue, and alleviate pain, making them effective in symptom management even before a conclusive diagnosis is made. This approach is often chosen when symptoms are severe and affect daily life, as waiting for surgery can delay relief. Another benefit of this option is that the medical treatments can slow the progression of endometriosis.

Additionally, a laparoscopy is an invasive procedure, so doctors may prefer to try non-invasive treatments first, especially if there's a strong suspicion of endometriosis based on clinical symptoms, family history, or imaging tests like ultrasound or MRI. Even if laparoscopy is eventually needed for confirmation, symptom relief through medical treatment can improve your overall well-being while awaiting further diagnostic evaluation.

Why does it take so long to get diagnosed?

Unfortunately, it still takes far too long to diagnose for several reasons. There is often not enough awareness about the condition. Also, because people consider painful periods to be part and parcel of being someone who menstruates, they may be dismissive and not take the concerns seriously to arrange investigations or referrals. Diagnosing endometriosis can also take years because the symptoms overlap with other common conditions like irritable bowel syndrome or ovarian cysts, leading to misdiagnosis or delay.

The other issue is that we don't have very good non-invasive tests; imaging tests like ultrasound and MRI scans can suggest endometriosis but can't confirm it. However, the gold standard for making a conclusive diagnosis is a laparoscopy, which has as its own costs, risks, and potential delays. These factors, combined with the variability in symptoms, mean many people wait 7–10 years before receiving a definitive diagnosis.

Will I be able to get pregnant if I have endometriosis?

Infertility or difficulty conceiving is a common symptom of endometriosis. Around 4 in 10 people who have endometriosis find it difficult to fall pregnant. Looking at the issue from another perspective, up to 50% of women who struggle with fertility have endometriosis.[7]

Although endometriosis can affect fertility in many different ways, there is a very broad spectrum. Some people do require fertility treatment to conceive, but others get pregnant easily without any issue.

Endometriosis can cause infertility through increased inflammation, which causes damage to developing eggs, or through scarring to the fallopian tubes. Whether your fertility is affected can depend on the severity of the endometriosis, and also where the endometriosis is located, such as if it blocks the fallopian tubes, or causes cysts on the ovaries.

The best way to check your fertility is when you actively try to conceive. If you know your endometriosis is severe and you haven't conceived after 6–12 months, your doctor can arrange tests to determine the next steps.

Are there good treatments for endometriosis?

Endometriosis treatments focus on relieving pain, reducing the growth of endometrial tissue, and improving fertility, as unfortunately we do not currently have an ultimate cure for this condition.

It can take time to find the right treatment with the maximum benefit, so we often begin trying treatments in this order, or in combination with each other:

- **Pain relief medications,** such as non-steroidal anti-inflammatory drugs (NSAIDs), can help alleviate pain and discomfort caused by endometriosis

- **Hormonal therapies**, such as the combined oral contraceptives, progesterone-only medications, and GnRH agonists are also commonly used. (More about each of these in Chapter 6 on contraception.) These treatments help manage symptoms by reducing or halting the menstrual cycle, which can limit the growth of endometrial tissue and reduce inflammation

- **Surgical treatments**, such as laparoscopic or robotic surgery, may be considered, to remove or destroy endometrial implants, which can provide relief from pain and improve fertility. In extreme cases, a hysterectomy (removal of the uterus) may be considered, although this is typically a last resort, especially for women who wish to preserve fertility

While these treatments can help manage pain and improve quality of life, endometriosis is a chronic condition, and symptoms may recur, requiring ongoing management and personalised care.

Fibroids

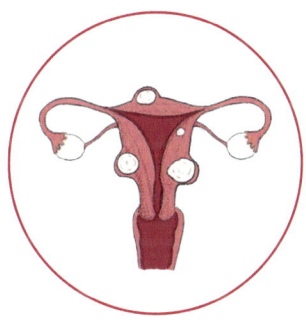

Fibroids are non-cancerous growths that develop in or around the uterus. They're made of muscle and fibrous tissue and can vary in size from very small to large. Many people with fibroids don't have any symptoms, but some may experience heavy periods, abdominal pain, a feeling of fullness in the lower abdomen, or frequent urination. Fibroids can also cause complications during pregnancy or affect fertility, though this is less common.

The prognosis for fibroids is generally good, as they are usually benign and often shrink after menopause. Fibroids can be treated with medication, such as hormonal therapies to help reduce symptoms like heavy bleeding and pain. In more severe cases, surgical options such as myomectomy (removal of the fibroids) or hysterectomy (removal of the uterus) may be recommended, depending on the size, location, and symptoms of the fibroids.

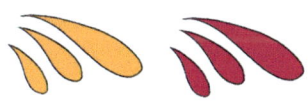

Ovarian cysts

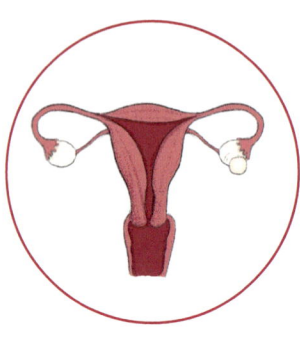

Ovarian cysts are fluid-filled sacs that develop on or inside the ovaries. Most ovarian cysts are benign and don't cause any symptoms, often disappearing on their own without treatment. To determine which cysts are benign and which might be problematic, doctors look at certain characteristics such as size, appearance, and complexity on imaging tests like ultrasounds. Simple cysts, which are fluid-filled and have smooth walls, are typically benign, while complex cysts that contain solid areas, thick walls, or irregular features might raise concerns for malignancy. Other factors like age, family history, and associated symptoms (e.g., pain or bloating) also play a role in assessing the risk.

Benign simple cysts can still be problematic as they can cause pain, bloating, or a feeling of pressure in the lower abdomen, especially if they become large, rupture, or twist (known as ovarian torsion). If a cyst is causing symptoms, or is particularly large, your doctor might recommend treatment, which usually involves laparoscopic (keyhole) surgery. The prognosis for ovarian cysts is generally good, as most are benign and resolve without complications.

Endometrial polyps

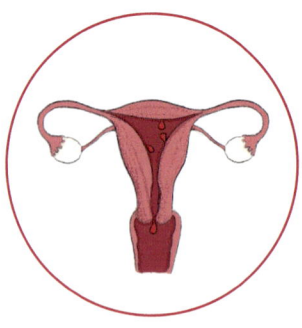

Endometrial polyps are small, soft growths that form on the lining of the uterus (endometrium). While many people with polyps experience no symptoms, others may have irregular spotting, bleeding between periods, or heavy menstrual bleeding. These polyps are usually benign (non-cancerous) but, in rare cases, they can become cancerous, which is why they are typically removed when detected. The outlook is generally positive, as polyps can often be removed through a simple procedure such as hysteroscopy, which involves inserting a small camera into the uterus.

PCOS

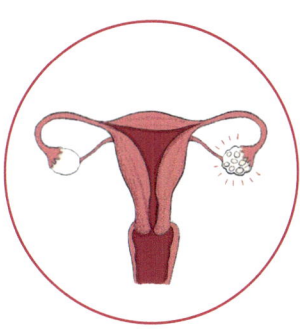

Polycystic ovary syndrome (PCOS) is a common condition affecting around 1 in 10 women and individuals with ovaries of reproductive age. It is characterised by a hormonal imbalance where the ovaries produce a higher-than-normal level of hormones called androgens (e.g., testosterone), which disrupts normal ovarian function. This often leads to the enlargement of the ovaries and the development of multiple small fluid-filled sacs, which is why it's called polycystic ovary syndrome.

Symptoms of PCOS can include irregular or absent periods, weight gain, acne, excessive hair growth on the face and body, and thinning hair on the scalp. The condition can also increase the risk of developing long-term health issues such as type 2 diabetes and heart disease.

Although there's no cure for PCOS, there are many options to help manage the condition and reduce its impact. Lifestyle changes, such as maintaining a healthy weight, eating a balanced diet, and regular exercise, can make a huge difference in improving the condition by regulating ovulation, which can make periods more predictable and improve fertility. Medications like hormonal contraceptives can also be used to control unpredictable periods and improve symptoms from raised androgen levels. For those struggling with fertility, specific medications can assist in stimulating ovulation. (More on this condition in the Chapter 4 on hormones!)

Pelvic Inflammatory disease

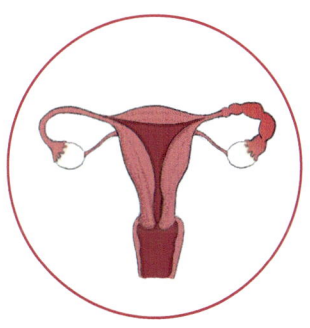

Pelvic inflammatory disease (PID) occurs when an infection spreads from the vagina or cervix to involve the rest of the pelvis, including the uterus, fallopian tubes, and ovaries. It is usually caused by bacteria from sexually transmitted infections (like chlamydia or gonorrhoea). Symptoms of PID can include lower abdominal pain, unusual vaginal discharge, fever, painful urination, and pain during sex.

If PID is caught early, it can be treated effectively with antibiotics, and most people recover fully. However, if left untreated, it can cause serious complications due to inflammation and scar tissue in the pelvis, which can affect fertility, cause ectopic pregnancy, and chronic pelvic pain. Prompt treatment is important for a good prognosis.

Check out Chapter 3 on sex for more!

FAQs

What happens to my periods if I am stressed?

Even when you don't realise you're stressed, your body does. Subtle changes in your stress levels lead to hormonal changes which can disrupt your menstrual cycle, sometimes causing your periods to become irregular, lighter, or even stop temporarily.

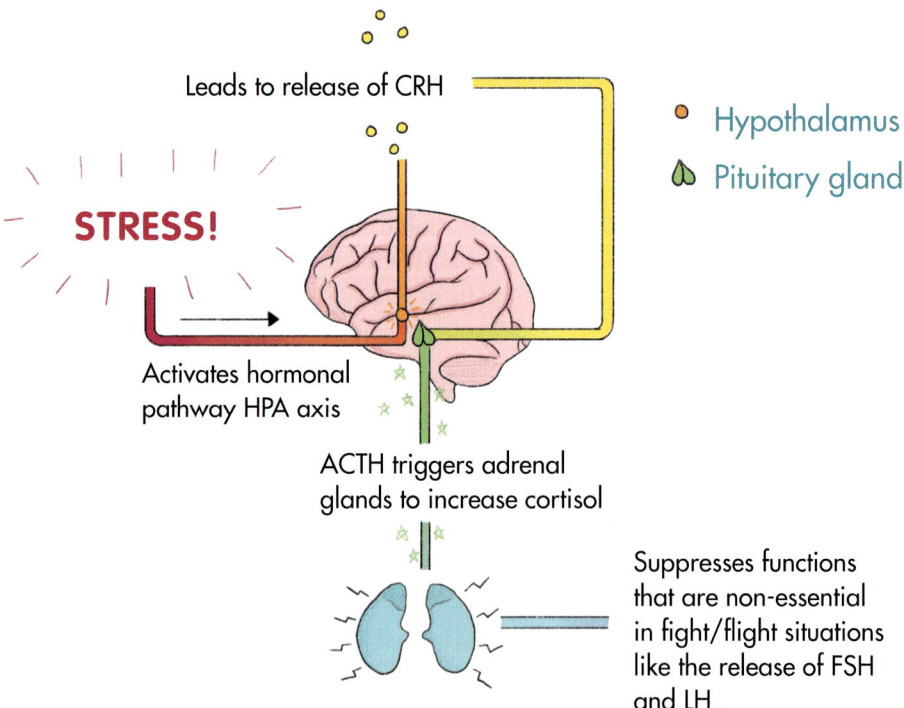

Leads to release of CRH

STRESS!

Hypothalamus
Pituitary gland

Activates hormonal pathway HPA axis

ACTH triggers adrenal glands to increase cortisol

Suppresses functions that are non-essential in fight/flight situations like the release of FSH and LH

When your brain perceives stress, subconsciously it activates the hormonal pathway called the hypothalamic–pituitary–adrenal (HPA) axis, which leads to the release of corticotropin-releasing hormone (CRH). This then stimulates the pituitary gland to produce adrenocorticotrophic hormone (ACTH), which triggers the adrenal glands to increase the levels of cortisol, the 'stress hormone'. Cortisol has many important roles in our body, like controlling our sleep cycles, blood pressure, blood glucose, and regulating metabolism. If your levels of cortisol rise, this not only affects your sleep cycles but also influences your menstrual cycles and libido. The HPA axis may be triggered by emotional stresses, such as having a busy time at work. You may also notice physical stresses can disrupt your periods such as when you are suffering with an illness, experiencing sudden weight loss, doing extreme exercise, or had a vaccination.

The idea is that it prepares our bodies for survival and suppresses any functions that would be non-essential in a fight-or-flight situation.

In your body, this can manifest as:

- Amenorrhea (no periods at all)
- Change in menstrual cycle length
- Irregular periods
- Worsening of premenstrual syndrome (PMS)
- Worsening of period pain

So, any type of stress, physical or psychological, can affect your period. This change is not usually permanent, so when that stress eases, the levels of hormones should regulate back to how they were before, and your menstrual cycle becomes predictable again.

Remember to track your cycles monthly so you are up to speed when any changes occur. A short-term change, where your periods are more irregular for a couple of months, should not be too worrying.

However, if you are worried, or the changes don't seem to improve once you try to change your lifestyle, check with your doctor to see if they can help!

What usually happens to periods as we get older?

As we age, periods often undergo several changes that are influenced by life stages, such as childbirth and the approach to menopause. Teenage years are often associated with unpredictable periods, but after the first couple of years of menstruating they usually become more regular and predictable. After childbirth, it's common for periods to be temporarily absent while breastfeeding and, when they return, they may initially be heavier or more irregular.

As you get older, some conditions such as endometriosis can progress if you are not on any treatment. This means that for some women and people who menstruate, periods can get more painful as the years go by. Fibroids are another condition that can progress, as they grow and respond to oestrogen over time, meaning periods can also get heavier over time.

As women approach menopause, typically in their 40s or 50s, periods often become irregular again, with cycles getting shorter or longer, and the flow may vary, with some very heavy and some lighter periods. Eventually, your periods will stop altogether, marking the onset of menopause. Hormonal fluctuations during these times can also impact symptoms like cramping and mood changes. (More on this in Chapter 9 on the menopause!)

Tests your healthcare professional may arrange

If you see your healthcare professional, such as a doctor or nurse practitioner, because of any concerns about your periods, they will begin by asking you many questions, so it is helpful to bring along a copy of your menstrual diary to aid the conversation. As well as talking about all of your symptoms, and your medical history, it is also important they ask about whether you are considering trying to conceive in the near future. This is because some of the common treatments for period concerns also act as contraception so this might sway which options you choose.

An examination of your pelvis is sometimes suggested if you are experiencing pain, abnormal bleeding, if you need a routine smear, or for a variety of other reasons. It should not be a routine part of every contact with the gynaecologist but it can add a lot of helpful information to this discussion.

What is a pelvic examination?

A pelvic examination usually involves your doctor feeling across your abdomen with their hands, to feel for any masses or to identify where you experience pain. They may also suggest an internal examination of your vulva and vagina.

If you are concerned about having a pelvic examination, discuss these feelings with your doctor or nurse so they can help put in place extra measures so you feel more comfortable. It is important to note that you do not have to have an internal examination, especially if you have never been sexually active or if you suffer from a condition like vaginismus. Instead, you can discuss alternatives to examination with your doctor.

For any intimate examination, you should be given a private space to undress and a blanket to cover yourself. The doctor should bring a chaperone with them. Usually, you would only need to undress from the waist down.

Once you are comfortable, you'll be asked to bend your legs and open them in what is known as a 'frog-legged' position. The doctor will put on gloves and examine the vulva to make sure that there are no sores or swellings. If required, the doctor will introduce a speculum to gently widen the view into the vagina. This is a thin piece of metal or plastic with a hinge on one end that allows it to open and close. Once the speculum is in the correct position, the doctor will gently open it up. That feeling can cause a bit of pressure and discomfort.

After the speculum is in place, the doctor or nurse will shine a light inside the vagina to look for anything unusual, like redness, swelling, discharge, or sores. The doctor may quickly wipe a cotton swab inside the vagina to collect a sample of mucus in order to test for infection, if necessary. The doctor will slide the speculum out as soon as the exam is done. This part of the exam only takes a minute or two.

The next part of the examination may involve the doctor examining the inside of the vagina using their finger while you stay in the same position. The doctor or nurse will put lubricant on two fingers (still wearing the gloves) and place them inside your vagina. Using the other hand, they may press on the outside of your lower abdomen (the area between your vagina and your stomach) and ask whether you experience any pain. You may feel a little pressure or discomfort. It can help if you focus on relaxing your pelvic floor muscles and taking slow, deep breaths.

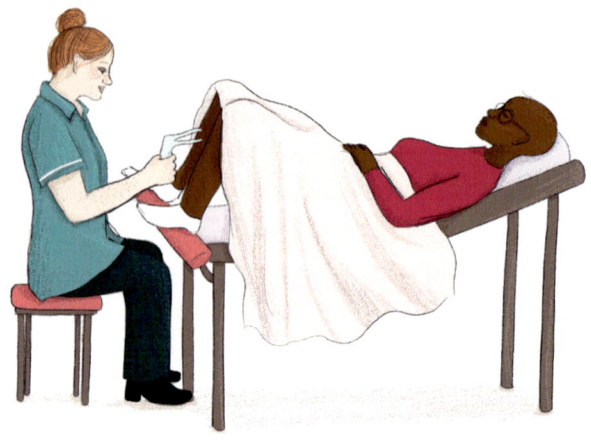

TOP TIPS FOR MAKING THE PELVIC EXAMINATION MORE COMFORTABLE:

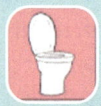

1. **EMPTY YOUR BLADDER:** Do this just before your appointment

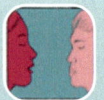

2. **TALK TO YOUR DOCTOR OR NURSE IF YOU'RE NERVOUS:** If you feel comfortable, share any history that is relevant, such vaginismus or previous sexual trauma

3. **ASK FOR A SMALLER SPECULUM:** Or ask to insert the speculum yourself

4. **GET READY:** Ask them to let you know just before the speculum is inserted

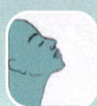

5. **USE YOUR BREATH:** Breathe out as the speculum is inserted

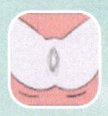

6. **TRY A DIFFERENT POSITION:** If you are not comfortable, ask to try a different position such as shifting your buttocks or placing your hands beneath the small of your back to elevate your pelvis

7. **DISTRACTION HELPS:** Use headphones to listen to music or meditation tracks, or try some simple breathing techniques to help you relax

What next?

Your doctor may then arrange some blood tests, such as checking your blood count and iron levels to see if you are anaemic, and testing your hormone levels.

After a physical examination they may also suggest further tests such as:

- Ultrasound scan

- Pelvic MRI scan

- Hysteroscopy

- Colposcopy

- Laparoscopy

What is an ultrasound scan?

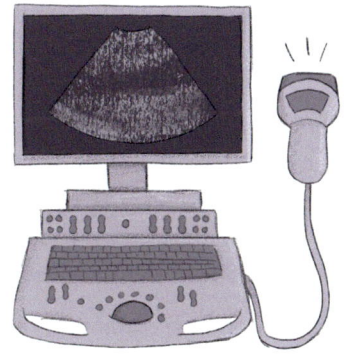

An ultrasound scan is a test that uses high-frequency sound waves (that you can't hear) to create an image of the inside of your body. Ultrasound scans are very safe and do not use X-rays.

A pelvic ultrasound may be transabdominal (through your lower abdomen) or transvaginal (from a probe placed within the vagina), or sometimes both in order to better visualise the uterus, ovaries, and cervix, as well as other organs like the bladder and bowels. Unlike static imaging such as X-rays, a gynaecological ultrasound is a dynamic, live test that allows the person performing the scan to observe the organs in real time. This means they can assess the movement, blood flow, and changes in the tissues, providing a detailed view that helps in diagnosing various conditions.

The probe will be covered in some gel to help produce a better-quality image. The ultrasound transducer (a small probe) is then moved slowly over your skin or within the vagina. Occasionally, they may need to press quite firmly in the area where you may be having pain. It is important to let the doctor or sonographer know if you feel uncomfortable at any point during the scan, especially as it may help them to understand where your pain is and look at that area more closely. You can ask them to stop at any point.

You may not be told immediately about the findings of the scan, as they may need to take some time to review the images and write a report. This is routine practice and doesn't mean there was anything wrong on the scan.

What is an MRI scan?

A pelvic MRI (magnetic resonance imaging) scan is a non-invasive imaging test that uses powerful magnets and radio waves to create detailed, accurate images of the organs and tissues in the pelvic region, including the uterus, ovaries, bladder, and surrounding areas. It is particularly useful for diagnosing and evaluating conditions like fibroids, endometriosis, pelvic tumours, and other abnormalities.

During the procedure, the patient lies on a table that slides into a large tube-like machine. The test is painless and provides high-resolution images, helping doctors make accurate diagnoses and plan treatments without the need for invasive procedures.

What is a hysteroscopy?

A hysteroscopy is a medical procedure used to examine the inside of the uterus. It involves a narrow telescope with a light and camera at the end called a hysteroscope. This is inserted through the cervix into the uterus, allowing the doctor to view the uterine lining directly on a screen.

This procedure is commonly used if you have an unusual bleeding pattern, or bleeding that occurs after the menopause. A hysteroscopy can be performed in a clinic or hospital, often under local or general anaesthesia, and can be both diagnostic and therapeutic, meaning that some conditions like fibroids or polyps can be treated during the same procedure.

What is a colposcopy?

A colposcopy is a medical procedure used to closely examine the vulva, vagina, and cervix for signs of disease. During the procedure, a special magnifying instrument called a colposcope is used to illuminate and magnify the area, allowing the doctor to identify abnormal cells or tissue more clearly. You may be referred for this investigation if you have had any unusual findings on a cervical screening result, or if there were any differences seen on your cervix at speculum.

The procedure is typically done in a clinic and doesn't require anaesthesia. If abnormal areas are found, the doctor may take a small tissue sample (biopsy) for further testing. A colposcopy is an important tool in the early detection and prevention of cervical cancer and other conditions.

What is a laparoscopy?

Laparoscopy is sometimes referred to as 'keyhole surgery' as it is a minimally invasive surgical procedure used to examine and treat conditions affecting the pelvis. During the procedure, a small incision is made usually starting at the belly button, and a thin tube with a light on the end of it, called a laparoscope, is inserted into the abdomen. Your abdomen is inflated with air, and then some additional small incisions will usually be made (no bigger than 0.5–1cm each) to allow the doctor to pass some instruments into the pelvis. This allows the doctor to view the organs on a screen and use the instruments to perform surgeries, like removing ovarian cysts, fibroids, or treating endometriosis, with precision.

Laparoscopy is often used for diagnosing unexplained pelvic pain, infertility, or other gynaecological issues and usually involves a quicker recovery time compared to open surgery.

Robotic surgery is another variation of laparoscopic surgery, as it is also 'keyhole' surgery. Instead, it uses advanced robotic systems to assist surgeons in performing minimally invasive procedures with greater precision and control. Despite the name, the robot doesn't operate independently; instead, the surgeon controls its movements from a console, ensuring every action is guided by human expertise.

Treatments your doctor may offer

After any tests are done, your doctor may discuss some options to help manage your symptoms. This may include general advice like painkillers, encouraging exercise and a healthy diet, which are all important in helping to regulate your cycle. The next steps may involve medication, such as hormonal treatments, or surgery depending on the nature of your concerns.

Usually, the first line of medications to try involves non-hormonal treatments such as painkillers, and some specific NSAID medications, which are similar to ibuprofen. One of these is called tranexamic acid and can be helpful to take on your heavy bleeding days as it can reduce the amount and duration of menstrual flow. Another option is mefenamic acid, which is a specific painkiller that can improve period cramps.

If those don't help, your doctor may talk you through some other choices, which usually involve hormonal medications such as combined hormones (which contain oestrogen and progesterone) or progesterone-only options. These come in various forms such as pills, implants, injections, patches, and coils so you can often find one to suit you! (Check out Chapter 6 on contraception for more on these different hormonal treatment choices!)

Depending on any underlying cause for your period concerns, such as if there is a suspicion of endometriosis, fibroids, or endometrial polyps, surgery might be the right choice for you. This might involve vaginal or abdominal surgery, and it might be an open or keyhole operation. Your healthcare team will be able to talk you through the different choices.

How to get the most out of your appointment

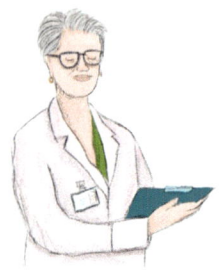

It can feel quite overwhelming if you know you are going to have an appointment to talk about your periods. Preparing well can help you to make the most out of the appointment. Here are some top tips to help you to advocate for yourself in a healthcare setting:

TOP TIPS FOR ADVOCATING FOR YOURSELF:

1. **MAKE A LIST OF QUESTIONS IN ADVANCE:** Have a think about how your symptoms are affecting your life

2. **BRING RECORDS:** Take along any records or letters from previous appointments and scans

3. **KEEP A MENSTRUAL DIARY:** Do this for at least a few months before your appointment. You can do this with an app on your phone, and it is helpful to record the days that you bleed but also how heavy they are, how much pain you have, and you can also record some of the symptoms you may have in the run-up to your periods if they are bothering you

4. **BRING A FRIEND:** It can be handy to bring with you a friend or family member so they can also listen and remember any parts of the consultation that you might have forgotten

5. **TAKE NOTES:** If you find it hard to remember what the doctor is saying, ask them to write down any key words for you so that you can look them up later, or ask if you can voice record a specific part of the consultation to listen to when you get back home

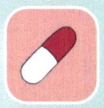

6. **ASK ABOUT SIDE EFFECTS:** If you are being prescribed any medication, ensure that you ask about any possible side effects or alternatives

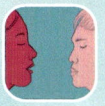

7. **ASK QUESTIONS:** Don't hesitate to ask questions if you're unsure about something!

Helpful questions to ask include:

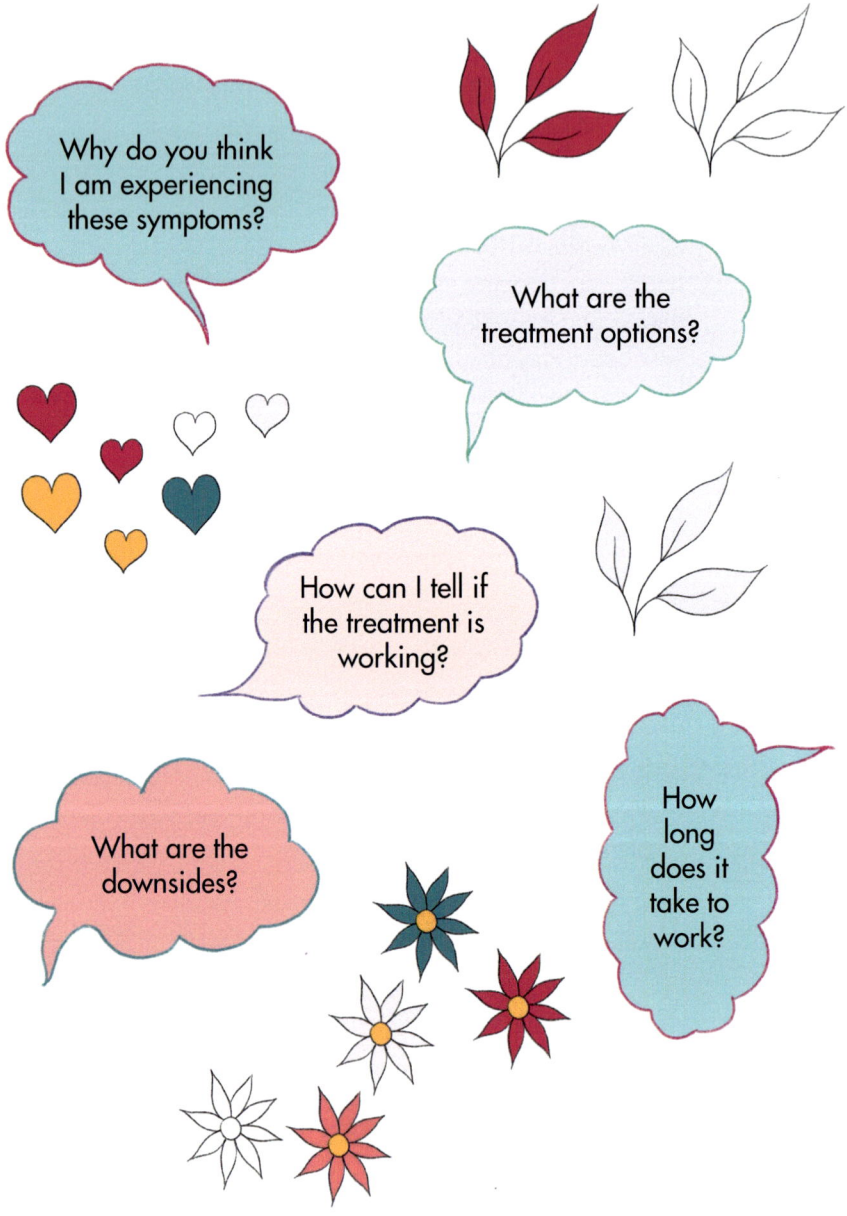

DID YOU KNOW?

- Tampons can't get lost! The end of the vagina is your cervix, so a tampon can't actually get lost although it can get tucked up behind the cervix and become difficult to reach

- Period blood can't flow when you are in a swimming pool! This happens because of the water pressure which holds the blood within the vagina. Often, you may become aware of a gush once you get out of the water once that water pressure disappears

- There is actually no evidence that you sync periods with your friends! While the idea of 'menstrual synchrony' (when women's cycles align when spending time together) is widely discussed, scientific evidence supporting this phenomenon is limited and controversial. Basically, there's a 25% chance each month you could be on at the same time, which is pretty high odds!

- Menstrual products have been used for centuries. Ancient civilisations used materials like wool, papyrus, and even sea sponges as primitive forms of tampons or pads

- Period pain is comparable to heart attack pain! This is why it is even more important to take period pain seriously, and never be afraid to speak up especially if it has a big impact on your quality of life!

Remember, every person's experience with periods is unique! The most important thing is to consider if your periods are having a significant impact on your life and investigating what can be done to help. By talking more about what we are each going through when it comes to periods, we can break some of the stigma and shame around menstruating and encourage each other to get help when it is needed!

Things to normalise during sex

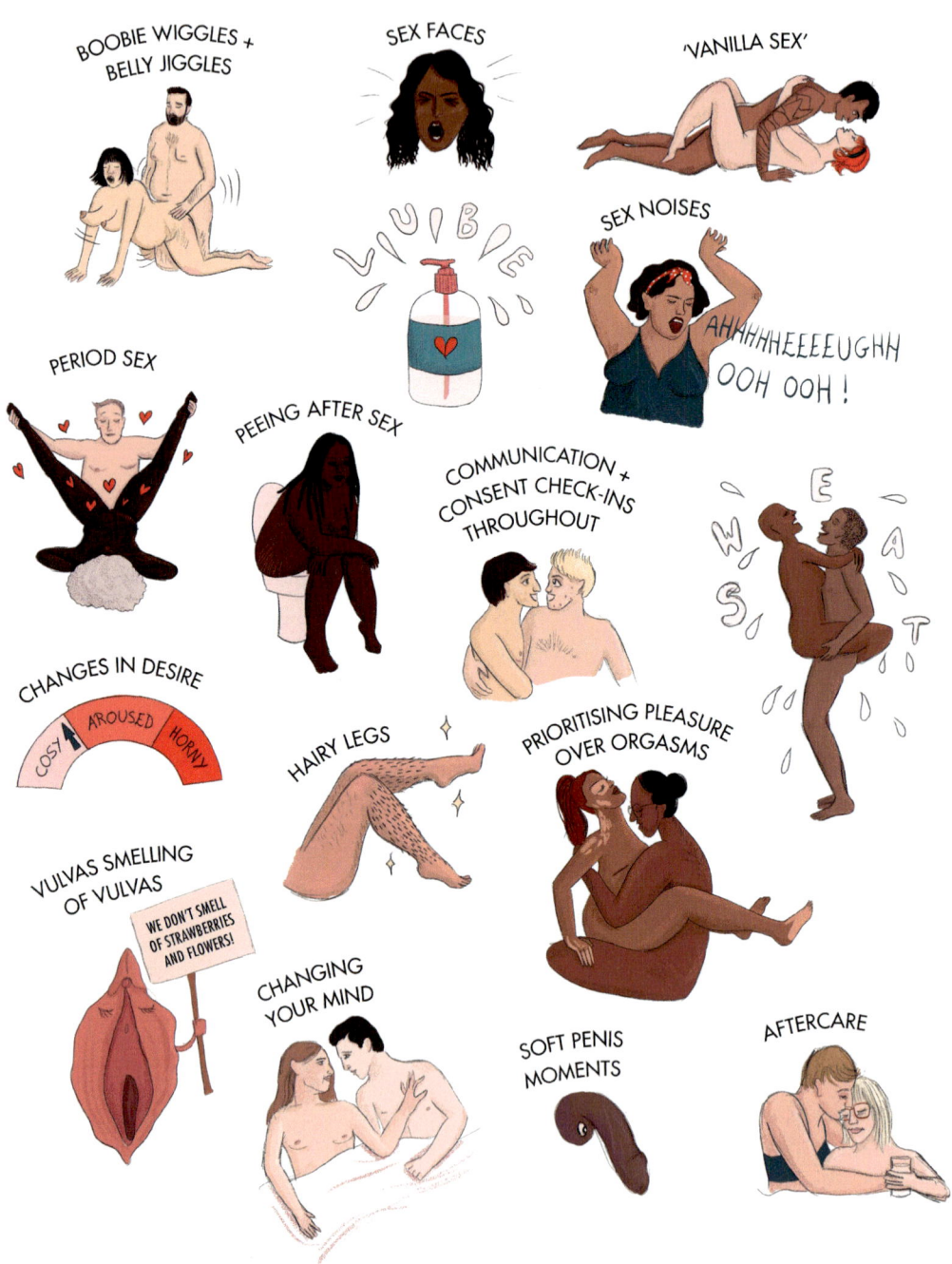

CHAPTER 3

Sex

Sex is a topic often surrounded by myths, misconceptions, and sometimes silence, yet it's an important part of pleasure, healthy relationships, and feeling comfortable in your body. Open conversations about sex allow us to understand what's typical, address concerns, and challenge stigmas.

What do we mean by the word 'sex'?

It is important to be aware that sex doesn't always mean penetration involving a penis and vagina! This description is often an oversimplification of a varied and complex practice. 'Sex' and 'intercourse' are not necessarily interchangeable terms, as they don't always mean the same thing. Many couples have meaningful and fulfilling sex lives which may not involve penetration at all. Sex is also not purely a physical act but involves psychological and social interactions, which are all interconnected.

Let's start with some definitions:

Sexual activity refers to a range of activities involving physical intimacy, often for the purpose of pleasure or reproduction. It includes various forms of sexual contact, such as vaginal intercourse, oral sex, anal sex, manual stimulation, and more.

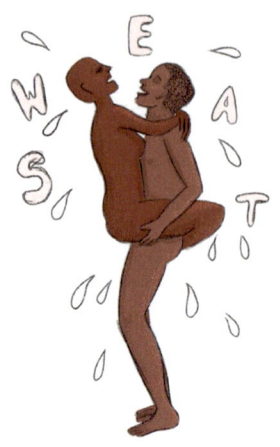

Sexual intercourse specifically refers to penetrative sexual activity, often involving the insertion of a penis into a vagina or, in the case of anal intercourse, the insertion into the anus. It can be between individuals of different or the same gender.

What is virginity?

Virginity is a concept that has been a part of many cultures and societies for a long time. It's a term that is used to describe someone who has not yet had their first sexual experience. It typically refers to a person's first experience of penetrative intercourse.

But here's the thing: virginity is a social and cultural idea, not a medical one. It means different things to different people and can be understood in various ways. Penetration alone can be difficult to define – is penetration with a tampon or finger the same? Does virginity only apply to penis-in-vagina sex? Some people believe the 'loss' of their virginity is a significant and meaningful moment in their lives, while others don't give it much thought. It's completely personal, and there's no right or wrong way to feel about it.

Now, let's talk about the **hymen**. The hymen is a thin, stretchy piece of tissue that partially covers the opening of the vagina. It's a part of a person's external genitalia. Contrary to what some might think, the presence or absence of a hymen isn't a reliable indicator of virginity. It also may surprise people to know that the hymen isn't usually a continuous piece of tissue, but it has a gap, or gaps, within it, which allows period blood to escape.

The hymen can vary in shape and size among individuals. It can be stretched or torn for various reasons that don't necessarily involve sex. Activities like sports, horseback riding, biking, or using tampons can cause the hymen to change or even tear. Some people are actually born with a hymen that has a more open structure, making it less likely to tear.

The idea that a person should bleed or experience pain during their first sexual encounter because of the hymen is a common misconception. While some people may experience minor discomfort, others may not feel much at all. Pain and bleeding during sex can happen for many reasons, including anxiety, lack of arousal, or a medical condition.

In conclusion, virginity is largely a social and cultural construct. The hymen, on the other hand, is a thin tissue near the vaginal opening that varies among individuals and isn't a reliable indicator of virginity. The idea of checking the hymen to know If someone is sexually active is utterly useless!

It's essential to remember that everyone's experiences are unique, and there's no one-size-fits-all definition of virginity. The most important thing is to make informed choices about your body and your sexual experiences that feel right for you, and prioritising communication, consent, and safety.

What is libido?

Libido is essentially a person's sexual spark – the drive or desire for intimacy and connection. It can show up in all sorts of ways: a sudden attraction, a lingering thought, or just that unmistakable feeling of wanting closeness. Libido isn't predictable or consistent; it can be shaped by everything from hormones and physical health to stress levels, relationship dynamics, and even a change in routine.

For instance, some people feel an increase in libido during ovulation or after a good workout, while others might notice it dips during busy or stressful times. Libido varies from person to person and can shift over time, which is completely natural. Additionally, libido can be influenced by a person's sexual orientation, their background. and personal preferences.

It's worth mentioning that having a high or low libido is not inherently indicative of a problem. It is more important that an individual's level of sexual desire aligns with their own feelings and comfort, and is respectful of any partners involved.

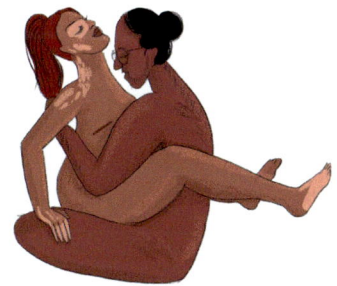

DID YOU KNOW?

Oestrogen plays a significant role in regulating libido (sex drive) as it can influence the production of neurotransmitters (chemical messengers) in the brain that are associated with sexual arousal and pleasure. Another important role of oestrogen for sex is that it promotes lubrication and elasticity in the vaginal area, which can enhance comfort and pleasure during sexual activity. It also increases sensitivity and can improve sexual pleasure and arousal.

Oestrogen levels vary throughout the menstrual cycle, meaning you might notice fluctuations in libido on a monthly basis. Levels usually peak with ovulation in the middle of the cycle, leading to a peak in libido.

Certain life stages also lead to lower levels of oestrogen, such as while breastfeeding or after the menopause. During these times it is natural to experience lower than typical libido.

Orgasm FAQs

What is an orgasm?

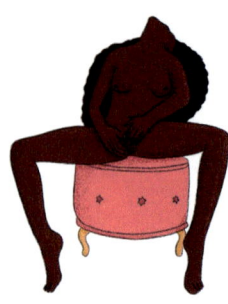

An orgasm is a complex mind–body reaction that indicates the peak of sexual arousal. It is characterised by intense pleasure, muscle contractions, and the release of hormones like oxytocin and endorphins. It involves a series of involuntary, rhythmic contractions of the pelvic muscles and can occur during various forms of sexual activity, including intercourse, oral sex, and self-stimulation.

Does everyone experience orgasm?

Not everyone experiences orgasm during sexual activity, and the likelihood of achieving orgasm can vary significantly between individuals.

One large US study reported that 95% of those who identified as heterosexual men reported experiencing orgasm regularly during sexual encounters, whereas only about 65% of those who identify as heterosexual women report the same consistency.[1] This discrepancy is often referred to as the 'orgasm gap'. It is believed to exist due to a combination of social, psychological, and anatomical factors.

One primary reason is that heterosexual encounters often prioritise vaginal intercourse, which doesn't always provide the clitoral stimulation many women need for orgasm. Additionally, cultural attitudes have historically emphasised male pleasure, leaving some women's needs less acknowledged or understood. Communication and connection with a partner play significant roles in sexual satisfaction and orgasm frequency.

For people with a vulva, the likelihood of orgasm can be influenced by the type of sexual activity, with clitoral stimulation being a key factor for many. Research has shown that 60–70% of women require clitoral stimulation to reach orgasm during sex.[2] There are other physical factors, such as low oestrogen and vaginal dryness, and emotional factors like stress and fatigue, which all contribute to whether an orgasm is achieved during sexual activity.

If we can improve our understanding of the orgasm gap and take steps to reduce it, we can empower women to feel comfortable expressing their sexual needs, enhancing satisfaction and intimacy for both partners.

Can you have an orgasm without penetration?

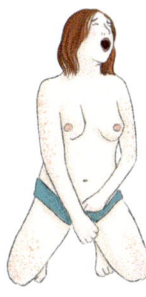

Yes, many people with a vulva achieve orgasm through clitoral stimulation alone, without any vaginal penetration. Orgasms can also be achieved through other forms of stimulation, such as oral sex, manual stimulation, or stimulation of other erogenous zones like the nipples.

Is it normal not to orgasm every time?

Yes, it's completely normal not to orgasm every time during sex. Many factors, like stress, emotional state, fatigue, and even the type of activity, can affect whether an orgasm occurs. More importantly, orgasm isn't the sole marker of good sex, nor should it be the goal. Enjoying the experience, feeling connected, and being present in the moment can be just as rewarding. Rather than racing towards an end point, focus on the journey itself – good sex is about mutual pleasure, connection, and exploration, not just reaching a climax.

Does the G-spot exist?

For decades, there has been debate about the existence of the 'G-spot'. Doubts around the existence of the G-spot stem from the difficulty in locating a specific anatomical structure that consistently produces sexual pleasure for all women. Unlike the clitoris, which is visibly identifiable and externally located, the G-spot is thought to be a sensitive area within the vaginal wall that may vary in sensitivity among individuals, making it challenging to define universally.

Some women report experiencing heightened sexual pleasure or orgasmic sensations when this specific area is stimulated, leading to the popularisation of the concept of the G-spot. However, scientific evidence on the G-spot is inconclusive.

Some researchers argue that the sensation associated with the G-spot may actually involve deeper structures like the clitoris, urethra, or even a combination of surrounding tissues, leading to differing experiences and definitions.

In summary, while some women experience enhanced sensitivity in a particular area inside the vagina, the G-spot remains a controversial and scientifically unverified concept. What is more important is that each owner of a vulva works out what feels good for them, rather than seeking a specific location!

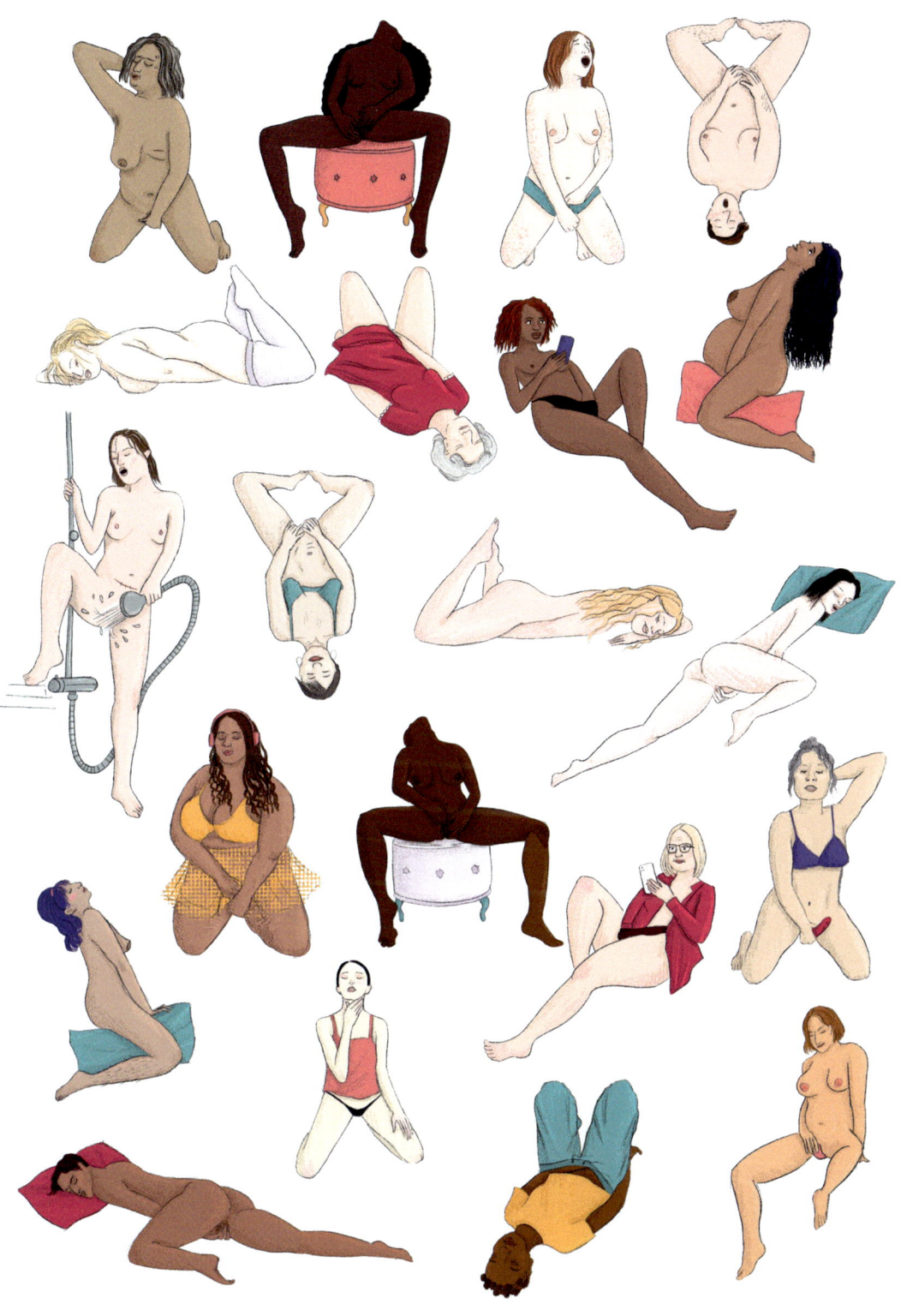

TOP TIPS FOR ENJOYABLE, SAFE SEX:

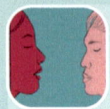 **1. COMMUNICATION:** Communication is the foundation of a healthy and safe sexual experience. It's like the secret ingredient that makes everything work better. Talk openly and honestly with your partner about your desires, boundaries, and any concerns you might have

- Don't be afraid to communicate during sex itself. Let your partner know what feels good, what doesn't, and if you'd like to try something different

- If you're experiencing any difficulties with arousal, pain, or satisfaction, talk to your partner about it. They may have insights or be able to provide support. Being worried about your partner realising you are in pain can often cause your pelvic floor to tighten more and worsen your discomfort. By sharing those worries you can work through options that could help, like a change in position or spending longer on non-penetrative forms of intimacy

- Frequency and timing: It can be really helpful to discuss your expectations regarding the frequency of sex and the best times for intimacy. Finding a balance that works for both of you is important. That doesn't mean sex needs to be scheduled, but being spontaneous may not be as easy when you lead busy lives. So, knowing you are on the same page can lead to better-quality sex even if the quantity may be less

- Feedback: Be open to giving and receiving feedback. Constructive feedback can help improve your sexual connection by letting your partner know what you love and what might need adjustment

- Safe sex and protection: Discuss safe sex practices, such as using condoms or other forms of contraception, and getting regular sexual health check-ups. Being responsible about sexual health benefits both of you after all!

- Remember that communication should be respectful, non-judgemental, and empathetic. It's about understanding each other's needs, desires, and boundaries while creating a safe and open space for sexual exploration and enjoyment

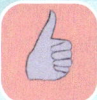

2. CONSENT: This should be the golden rule of sexual activity. Always check in with each other for consent, even if you've been together for a while. It means that all parties involved do willingly and enthusiastically agree to engage in sexual activity. Consent should be an ongoing conversation, and can be withdrawn at any time. It should be clear, specific, and never assumed. Always respect your partner's boundaries, and never pressure or coerce them into anything they're not comfortable with

Freely given
Reversible
Informed
Enthusiastic
Specific

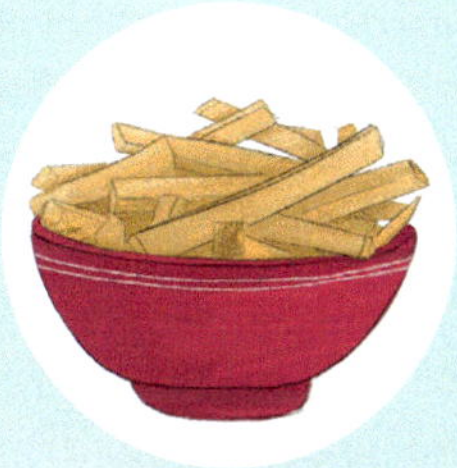

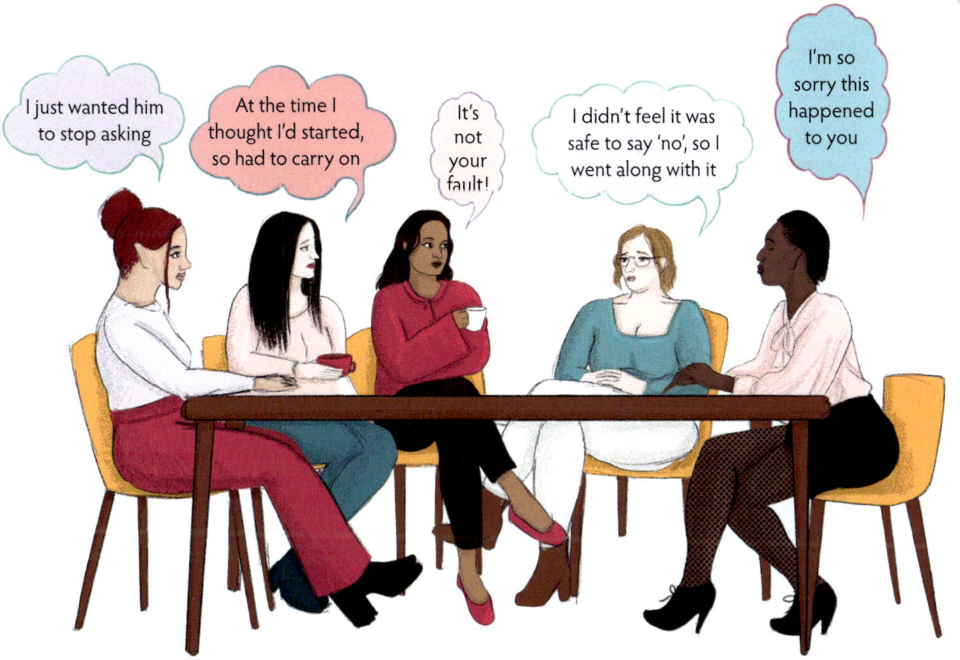

continued...

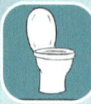

3. PEEING AFTER SEX: Peeing after sex might sound like an odd tip, but it's actually pretty important. After sexual activity, especially penetrative sex, it's a good idea for both partners (but especially those with vaginas) to urinate. This helps flush out any bacteria that might have entered the urethra during sex, reducing the risk of urinary tract infections (UTIs)

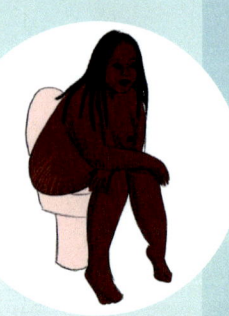

4. LUBRICATION: Lubrication is like the unsung hero of safe and pleasurable sex. It reduces friction, making sex more comfortable and less likely to cause irritation or small tears. Whether you're using condoms or not, adding some water-based or silicone-based lubricant can enhance the experience. If you're not producing enough natural lubrication (which can happen for various reasons), don't hesitate to introduce lubrication to keep things smooth and enjoyable. It is also very important to know that using lube doesn't mean you are not aroused!

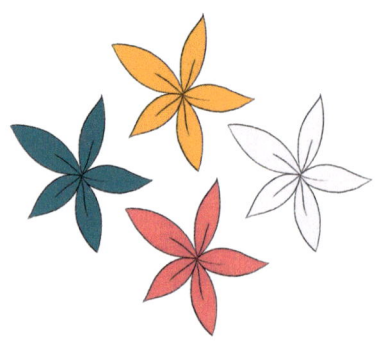

Painful sex – is it ever normal?

Sex is supposed to be an enjoyable and exciting experience but sometimes that isn't the reality. In fact, around 10–20% of women experience painful sex at some point.[3] Painful sex, while common, is not 'normal' and shouldn't be dismissed.

Sometimes, pain during sex can be temporary and may resolve on its own, such as when caused by occasional dryness or tension. In these cases, it's not necessarily a sign that something more serious is wrong. However, if the pain is recurring or impacting enjoyment and intimacy, it's worth discussing with a healthcare provider. Even if it's a common experience, painful sex shouldn't be trivialised, as support and effective treatments are available to help address it and improve comfort and quality of life.

There are many causes of painful sex. Let's explore the common ones.

The most common cause? Vaginal dryness

Sex is always better when lubricated! Nearly half of women who report pain during sex have also noticed vaginal dryness.[4] If your vagina is as dry as the desert and you try to put something inside, you'll likely experience discomfort or even feel like you're getting a friction burn.

Vaginal dryness is usually associated with a drop in a hormone called oestrogen. This is why it is more common if you are breastfeeding, or around the menopause, when there is a natural drop in the levels of this hormone.

If you are experiencing vaginal dryness, it could be time to embrace the lube! Using a small amount of lubricant before sex can make the experience more pleasant and less painful, and shouldn't just be reserved for post-menopause! Ideally, everyone should use lubricant for all sexual encounters!

For more persistent dryness, using vaginal moisturisers regularly can help improve hydration and elasticity. Vaginal oestrogen therapies (available as creams, tablets, or rings) are safe and effective, and can be used on a regular basis to target the oestrogen delivery to replace it where it is needed in the vagina, with minimal absorption into the bloodstream.

Superficial pain

Other than dryness, there are a number of reasons why sex can hurt, both during or after the act. Your doctor may ask whether you experience the pain inside your vagina, or deeper in your pelvis. If your pain is superficial, involving mainly the vulva or in the lower part of the vagina, it may be caused by:

- **Infections:** These may include thrush or a sexually transmitted infection (STI) like chlamydia or genital herpes
- **Skin conditions:** These include conditions such as psoriasis and lichen sclerosis, or allergies to things like latex condoms, soap products, or spermicides
- **Vulvodynia:** This is a chronic pain condition that causes burning, stinging, or irritation of the vulva. It may be triggered by activities like sexual intercourse, sitting for long periods, or wearing tight clothes. The exact cause isn't well understood, but it may be related to nerve issues, hormonal changes, or past trauma
- **Vaginismus:** This is a condition which involves a mind–body reaction to stimulation, which causes the muscles around the vagina to involuntarily tighten or spasm, making penetration difficult, painful, or sometimes impossible. This can occur during sexual intercourse, a pelvic exam, or when inserting a tampon. The exact cause can vary, but it may develop in response to past infections, anxiety, or a history of sexual trauma

Pain felt within the entire pelvis

If the pain that you experience occurs on deeper penetration, or is felt in your pelvis or abdomen rather than the vagina, your pain may be caused by conditions that affect your internal organs such as the uterus and bowel. While these conditions cause pain during sex, they usually have other telltale signs and symptoms so it's important to take note of anything else that seems abnormal.

If your pain during sex is coming from your pelvis, it may be caused by conditions such as:

- Endometriosis

- Fibroids

- Ovarian cysts

- Adhesions from previous pelvic surgery or infections

- Pelvic inflammatory disease (PID)

- Constipation

- Irritable bowel syndrome (IBS)

Psychological causes of painful sex

Vaginismus is a mind–body response to the fear of vaginal penetration – the vaginal muscles tighten involuntarily, making penetration impossible or very painful. This can prevent penetration during intercourse either completely or partially, and causes pain which can even feel sharp like razor-blades.

Other symptoms of vaginismus include:

- Not being able to have penetrative sex or insert a tampon at all

- Fear or anxiety about vaginal penetration

- Loss of sexual desire

For some women with vaginismus, the debilitating symptoms may begin early in puberty, when they first attempted to insert a tampon, or around the time of a painful first experience of sex. This is known as primary vaginismus.

Vaginismus can, however, also occur after vaginal function has been normal for many years This is called secondary vaginismus. Vaginismus can occur intermittently – in certain contexts and circumstances only – so it can come and go throughout your lifetime.

There are many potential triggers that can lead to vaginismus including:

- A previous experience of sexual trauma

- Other vaginal trauma such as childbirth

- A history of urinary or vaginal infections

- Stress and anxiety

- Cultural stigma suggesting shame or embarrassment associated with sex
- Issues surrounding body image

What should you do if you experience pain with sex?

Sex should be an enjoyable experience and can be an important part of a relationship; you shouldn't have to suffer in pain through it. If pain persists, it's important to ring your GP or a healthcare professional at a sexual health clinic. They'll be able to check you over and recommend any treatment options depending on your symptoms.

To help your medical team and yourself to work out what may be going on, you can ask yourself some questions:

- **What kind of pain are you experiencing?** Is it a stabbing pain, burning sensation, or a niggling pain?
- **Where is the pain coming from?** Does the pain feel like it's deep inside your pelvis or superficial?
- **When do you experience the pain?** Does the pain come during penetration or is it associated with certain positions?

These questions can help determine the most likely cause, as a stabbing deep pain may be suggestive of endometriosis, whereas a burning superficial pain may represent vaginismus.

Depending on the cause of your pain, your doctor may suggest medications for an infection, using vaginal lubricants and moisturisers, stopping use of fragranced body care products, taking a form of oestrogen replacement or treatment for emotional issues at the root of the problem.

If your pain relates to vaginismus, treatment may also involve referral to a psychosexual therapist or a pelvic health physiotherapist.

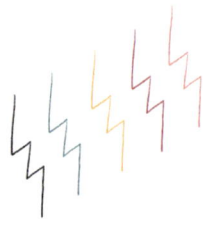

Recipe for enjoyable, safe sex

INGREDIENTS

- Lube
- Communication
- Consent
- Pleasure
- Optional: sex toys, music, pirate hat, etc.

Feel free to play with your levels of spice, from vanilla to extra spicy

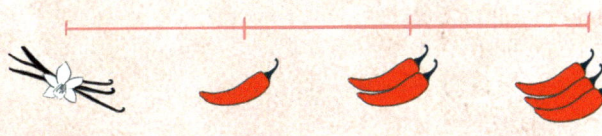

METHOD

1. PREPARATION GETS THE BEST RESULTS

Communicate freely, explore your desires and concerns so that you know your partner is on the same page. Talk about what you enjoy and what doesn't work for you.

Sometimes taking penetration off the table can allow you to enjoy an intimate experience with your partner without feeling stressed or pressurised

2. EXPLORE AND ENJOY!

New positions, new lubes, new toys: explore new things to find better and wetter positions! Nobody should need a reason to use lubricant; it should be part of everyone's routine practice for any type of sex. You may also find adding in more time spent on foreplay or different positions for sex can help increase arousal, reducing tension, and improving your pain

3. BE EASY ON YOURSELF

Sex is supposed to be fun and there can be a lot of pressure to pretend you're okay. You can't force yourself to have a good time and it's important to be honest with your partner about what is going on

STIs and protecting yourself

Sexually transmitted infections (STIs) are common, and absolutely nothing to be ashamed of. We need to normalise talking about these conditions so we can also appreciate the importance of practising safe sex!

STIs are infections that are primarily spread through sexual contact, including vaginal, anal, or oral sex. Common STIs include chlamydia, gonorrhoea, syphilis, herpes, human papillomavirus (HPV), HIV, and trichomoniasis, among others.

Some STIs are caused by bacteria, while others are caused by viruses or parasites.

If you're sexually active and don't have a long-term partner, getting a sexual health screen every 6 months should be a routine, normalised part of your self-care. Many STIs don't show symptoms, so you could have one without even knowing it – but a simple screen helps you catch and treat infections early. Regular screening isn't just about protecting your health; it's about feeling confident and empowered in your sex life, knowing you're looking after yourself and any future partners.

Common symptoms of STIs in women and people with a vagina may include:

- Unusual vaginal discharge, which may be yellow, green, or have an unpleasant smell
- Pain or discomfort during urination or sex
- Itching or burning in the genital area
- Sores, blisters, or warts in the genital or anal area
- Abnormal bleeding between periods or after sex
- Pelvic pain or lower abdominal pain

Testing methods vary depending on the STI but may involve blood tests, urine samples, vaginal swabs, or physical examinations. A lot of these tests can be less invasive these days, and they may be available as self-testing kits rather than needing to have a doctor or nurse take the samples for you. If you are worried about having the tests, it is better to have an appointment to discuss the different options so the nurse or doctor can help you feel more comfortable on the day!

Different treatment options for STIs will be offered depending on the type of infection. Common treatments include the following:

- **Antibiotics:** Bacterial STIs like chlamydia, gonorrhoea, and syphilis are often treated with antibiotics

- **Antiviral medications:** Viral infections like herpes and HIV are managed with antiviral drugs. While there's no cure for herpes, antivirals can help treat symptoms and reduce how often outbreaks happen

- **Vaccination:** HPV vaccines are available to protect against certain strains of the virus that can lead to cervical cancer and genital warts

Make sure to complete any prescribed courses of medication, even if symptoms improve to ensure the infection is really gone for good!

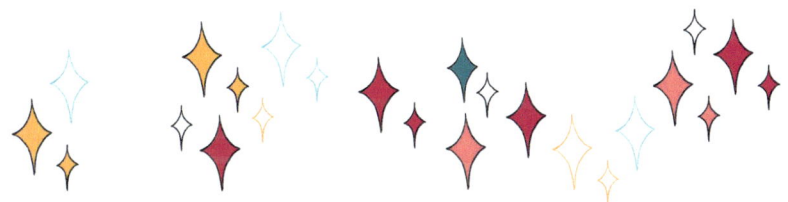

How can you reduce the chances of catching an STI?

- Remember that hormonal contraception only protects against pregnancy and not STIs! Practise safe sex by using barrier methods like condoms

- Open the conversation about sexual health with any new partner, and encourage them to get tested before becoming intimate if possible

- Get vaccinated against preventable STIs (e.g., HPV)

Early detection and treatment are crucial for managing STIs effectively and preventing complications like pelvic inflammatory disease. It is important not to delay your visits to a sexual health clinic so you can limit any long-term effects!

There are several common myths and misconceptions about (STIs):

MYTH 'You can't get an STI if you're in a monogamous relationship'

FACT While being in a monogamous relationship reduces the risk of STIs, it doesn't guarantee immunity. Some STIs can actually lie dormant in your body for a number of years before becoming apparent. If you develop an STI in a monogamous relationship it doesn't always mean your partner had an affair!

MYTH 'You'll know if you have an STI because there will be obvious symptoms'

FACT Many STIs, including chlamydia, gonorrhoea, and HPV, often have no noticeable symptoms, especially in the early stages. Regular testing is crucial for accurate diagnosis and treatment.

MYTH 'Only "promiscuous" or "irresponsible" people get STIs'

FACT Anyone who is sexually active can contract an STI, regardless of their relationship history or number of partners.

MYTH 'You can't get an STI from oral or anal sex'

FACT STIs can indeed be transmitted through oral, anal, as well as vaginal sex. Some infections, like herpes, HPV, chlamydia, and gonorrhoea, can be contracted through various sexual activities.

MYTH 'You can't get the same STI twice'

FACT While some STIs, like herpes, can become dormant and reactivate, it's possible to be re-infected with the same or a different strain of an STI.

MYTH 'If you're using birth control, you don't need to worry about STIs'

FACT Birth control methods, such as pills, patches, and intrauterine devices, do not provide protection against STIs. Condoms are the most effective barrier method for preventing their transmission.

MYTH 'You can't transmit an STI if you've been treated and the symptoms have gone away'

FACT Even after successful treatment, some STIs can still be present in the body, and potentially could be transmitted to a partner. A test of cure after treatment is often recommended.

MYTH 'STIs only affect young people'

FACT STIs can affect individuals of all ages. Rates of STIs have been increasing among older adults in recent years.

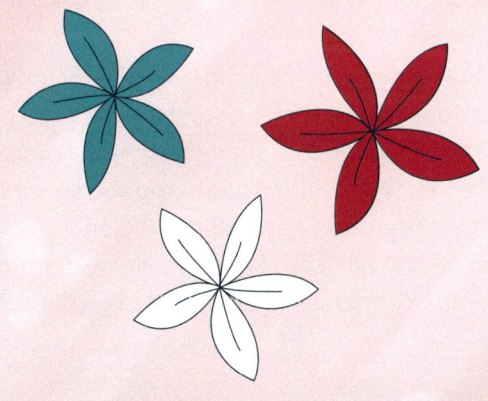

What do the different colours of discharge mean?

Have you ever noticed the rainbow of different colours that can emerge from your vagina throughout your cycle? Checking the colour and texture of vaginal discharge can give you lots of clues about the well-being of your vagina and hormones. Discharge naturally changes throughout the cycle due to hormone shifts, and a range of colours and textures can be normal. However, some unusual changes may signal an infection, so it's helpful to be familiar with your body's patterns and recognise when something feels different.

While checking vaginal discharge can give some insight into your menstrual cycle and reproductive health, focusing too much on its colour can be misleading. Discharge varies naturally due to hormonal shifts, diet, stress, and even exercise, and these variations don't necessarily signal a problem.

Let's take a closer look.

Menstrual cycle

- **Menstrual phase:** Discharge appears as blood (red or brown) and may have some clotting. Heavier bleeding tends to pass out more quickly, so the heavier the flow, the redder the blood will look and it may also contain some lumps known as 'clots' (have a look at Chapter 1 – page 27 for more).

  Dark red blood is also normal, especially in the morning after lying down, as the blood collects and oxidises in the uterus overnight. Dark red blood is often seen towards the end of a period or after giving birth (known as 'lochia'). Brown or black blood is simply older, more oxidised blood that has taken longer to leave the body, often appearing at the end of your period or with a slower flow. Although it can look alarming, black blood is usually just very old blood and is generally not a sign of a health problem.

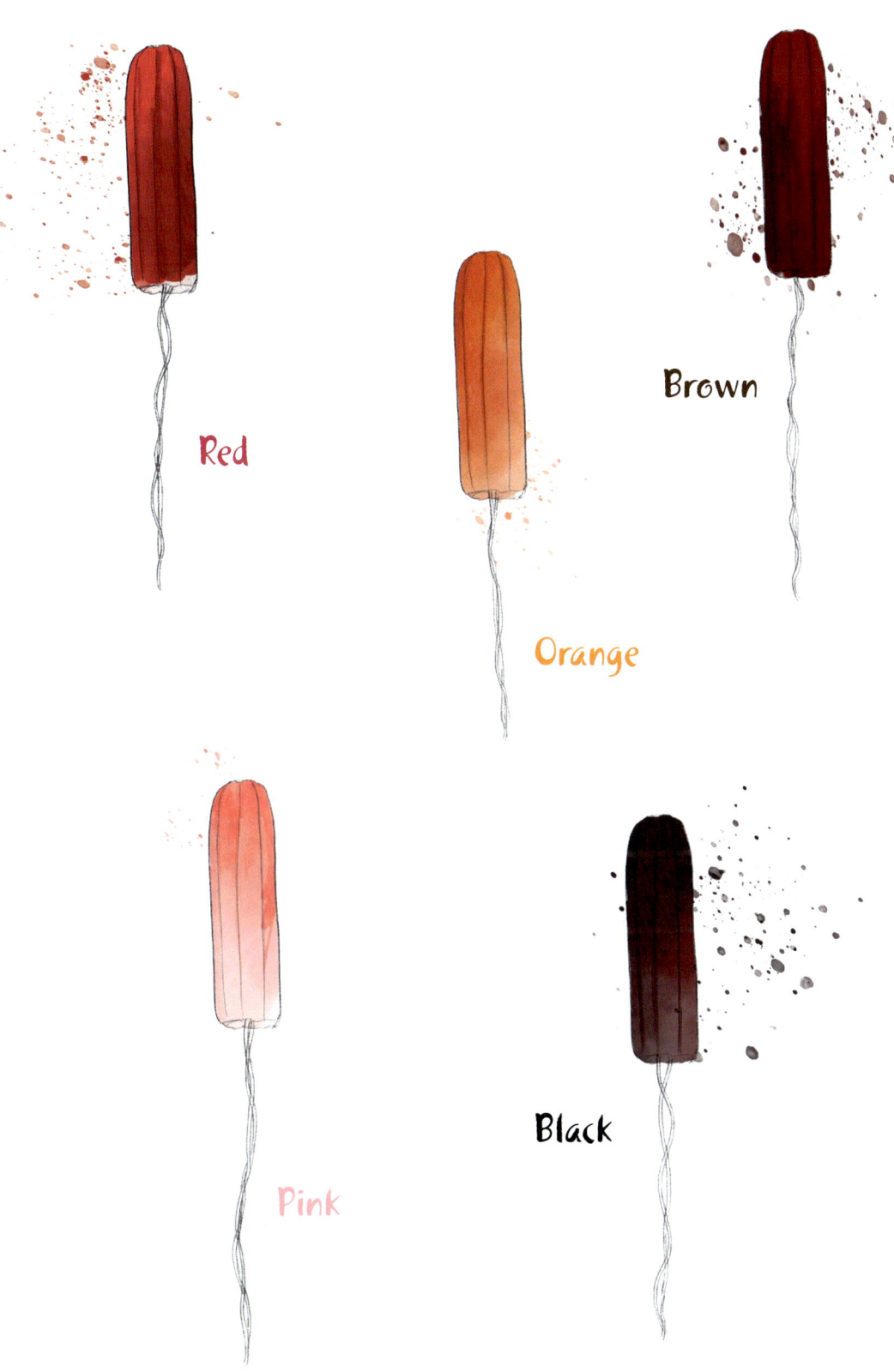

Red

Brown

Orange

Pink

Black

Period blood can take on a pink tint when it mixes with cervical fluid, which can sometimes happen at the start or end of your period as your discharge changes and dilutes the blood. You might also experience pink bloody discharge after sex, as sometimes intercourse can leave you with small tears in the vagina or cervix that heal on their own. Blood from these tears mixes with fluid in your vagina and leaves the body looking like pink discharge. However, it is important that you don't ignore bleeding after sex as it can sometimes occur if there's a more sinister underlying cause like cervical cancer.

See pages 25–29 for more about what to expect from discharge at each stage of the menstrual cycle.

Infections

- **STIs:** Some STIs, like chlamydia or gonorrhoea, may cause yellow or green discharge, often accompanied by a strong odour or pain. However, not all infections show symptoms

- **Bacterial vaginosis (BV):** Discharge may become greyish and thin or watery, with a strong fishy odour, especially after sex. This may indicate a common infection called BV. It is not sexually transmitted, but occurs due to a change in the balance of bacteria in the vagina, and can be treated with antibiotics

- **Thrush (yeast infection):** If you notice thick, white, and clumpy discharge, which may bear resemblance to a spoon-full of cottage cheese, you may have a fungal infection known as candida, or thrush. This discharge may also be accompanied by itching or irritation and again, is not transmitted sexually but rather occurs due to changes in the balance of the microbiomes in the vagina. It can be treated with antifungal medications

Ultimately, when it comes to your discharge you should get to know what is normal for you at different times of your cycle. If you notice any changes or something just doesn't seem right, chat to your doctor to see if they recommend any further tests.

Understanding what you can expect from sex, from orgasm and libido to whether pain can ever be normal, is vital for fostering a healthy relationship with your body and your partner. Knowledge empowers you to recognise any changes, address concerns, and improve communication about intimacy. Whether it's exploring pleasure, identifying sources of discomfort, or simply becoming more informed, these insights are key to breaking down stigmas and building a more confident, satisfying, and informed approach to sexual health.

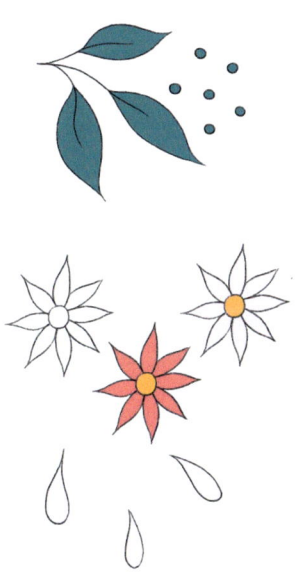

Hormones got me like...

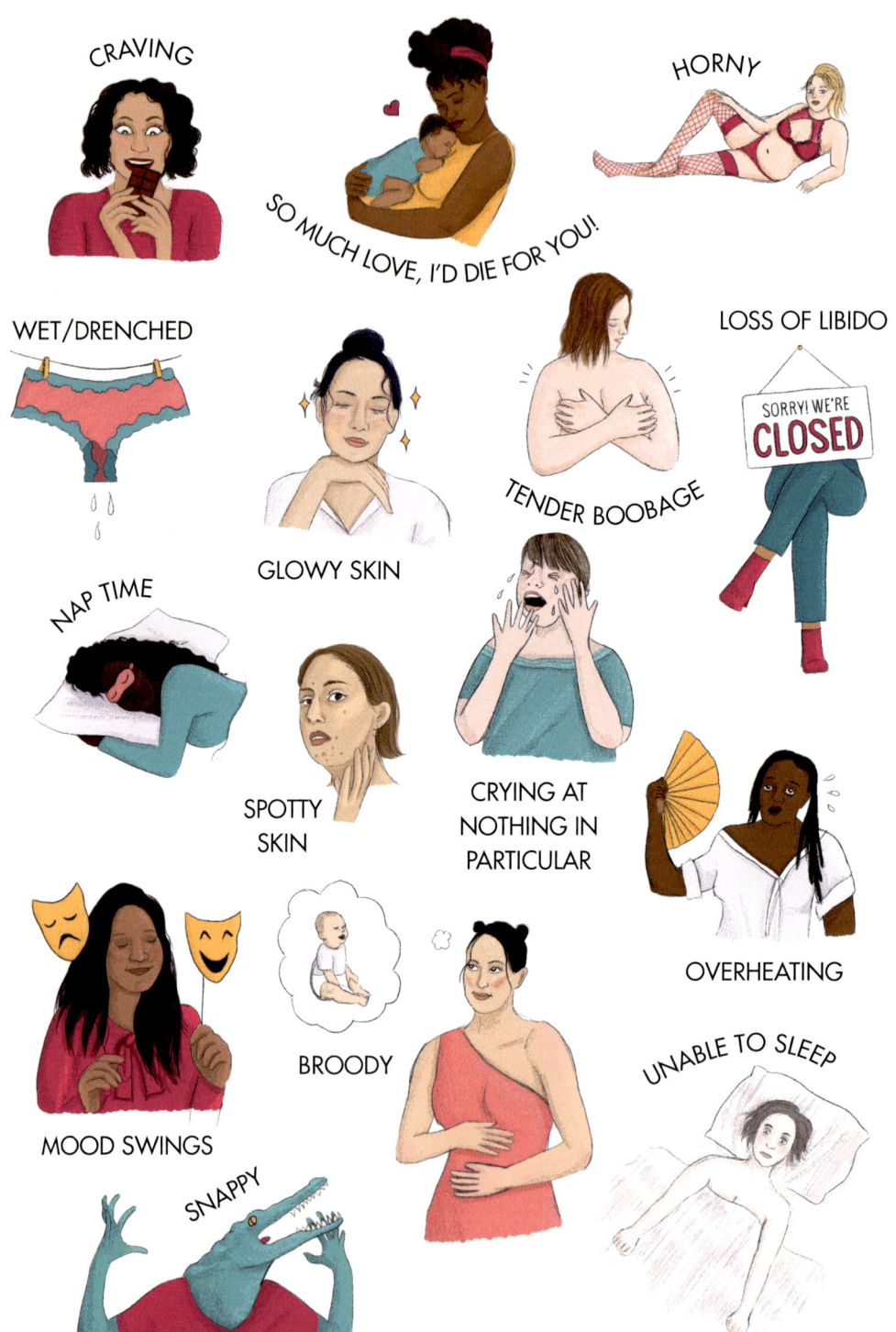

CHAPTER 4

Hormones:
what are they and why do they matter to me?

Hormones are chemical messengers, and so much of what happens in our bodies can be attributed to these molecules. If you are wondering how hormones work as messengers, it's actually pretty clever! The hormone travels through the bloodstream, acting like a key designed to fit into specific receptors on target cells. Once it binds to the receptor – its 'lock' – it triggers a chain reaction within the cell, instructing it to perform a specific function. This process allows hormones to regulate a wide variety of activities in the body, from controlling blood sugar levels to preparing the uterus for pregnancy or even influencing mood and energy.

When it comes to the menstrual cycles, there are several key players, but probably the most important are oestrogen and progesterone.

Oestrogen

Oestrogen is not exclusive to women and people who have ovaries. People who are post-menopausal, those who have a difference of sexual development (DSD), anyone transgender, as well as children, and men also have oestrogen in their bodies. In these people who may not be actively releasing eggs from their ovaries every month, their oestrogen is made in other areas of the body, such as in fat tissues, bones, skin, liver, and the adrenal gland. In adult men, oestrogen is produced in the testes.

Sources of oestrogen

Oestrogen is produced in various parts of the body at different life stages:

1. **Ovaries:** The main source of oestrogen during the reproductive years, especially oestradiol

2. **Adrenal glands:** Produce small amounts of oestrogen (especially oestrone) throughout life

3. **Fat tissue:** Converts androgens into oestrogen, especially important after menopause when ovarian production stops

4. **Placenta:** Becomes a temporary but powerful source of oestrogen during pregnancy

5. **Testes:** In smaller amounts, oestrogen is also produced in men and people with testes

What does oestrogen do?

Oestrogen, also spelled estrogen, is a group of hormones that play several important roles in the body. These include:

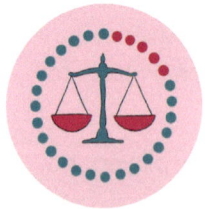

1. **Regulation of the menstrual cycle:** Oestrogen is the main hormone responsible for regulating the menstrual cycle. It helps to stimulate the growth of follicles, encourages ovulation to occur and it also helps prepare the uterus for potential pregnancy

92

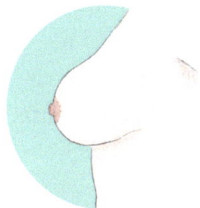

2. **Development of secondary sexual characteristics:** During puberty, oestrogen promotes the development of physical features such as breasts and the way body fat is distributed

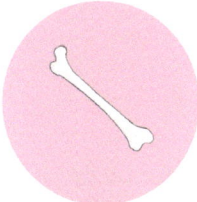

3. **Bone health:** Oestrogen helps to maintain healthy bones by preventing the breakdown of bone tissue. It is crucial for preventing conditions like osteoporosis

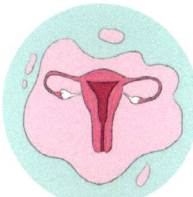

4. **Lubrication of vaginal tissues:** Oestrogen helps to keep the tissues of the vagina healthy and lubricated. This is important to avoid discomfort as well as improving experience of sex by reducing friction

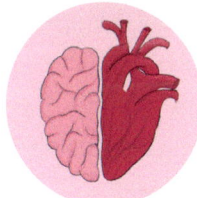

5. **The heart and brain:** We are starting to understand more about how oestrogen plays a protective role in heart and brain health by helping to keep blood vessels flexible and supporting healthy blood flow. Oestrogen helps to maintain healthy levels of 'good' cholesterol (HDL) and reduce levels of 'bad' cholesterol (LDL). Therefore, it also has a protective effect on the cardiovascular system. In the brain, oestrogen supports cognitive function, potentially protecting against the future development of dementia. This is still an area where more evidence is emerging all the time

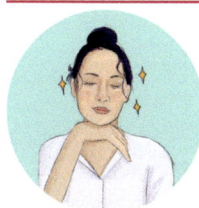

6. **Skin health:** Oestrogen contributes to the maintenance of skin elasticity and hydration

A lack of oestrogen in the body, which can occur in certain medical conditions as well as during breastfeeding and after menopause, can lead to a number of symptoms. These might include vaginal dryness, lower libido, or disrupted sleep. We talk more about these in Chapter 9 on the menopause, and what can be done to improve them.

Progesterone

What does progesterone do?

Progesterone is an important hormone that helps to prepare the body for pregnancy each month by nourishing the thickened lining of the uterus.

Sources of progesterone

1. **Corpus luteum:** After ovulation, when an egg is released from a mature follicle, the empty follicle transforms into the corpus luteum. This becomes a temporary gland which secretes progesterone, along with some oestrogen. If pregnancy doesn't occur, the corpus luteum will disappear again and a new one is made after the next ovulation

2. **Placenta (during pregnancy):** If fertilisation occurs and a pregnancy is established, the placenta takes over the production of progesterone to support the developing embryo and maintain the uterine lining

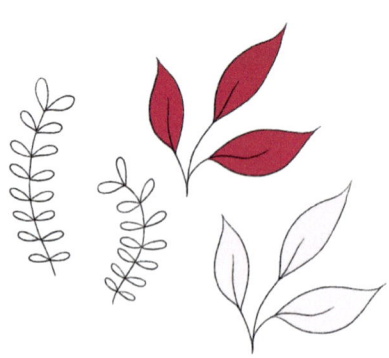

Functions of progesterone

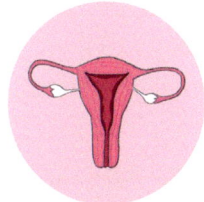

1. **Uterine lining support:** One of the primary functions of progesterone is to maintain the thickened uterine lining (endometrium) that developed during the first half of the menstrual cycle in response to oestrogen. This thickened lining provides a nourishing environment for a potential embryo to implant and establish a pregnancy

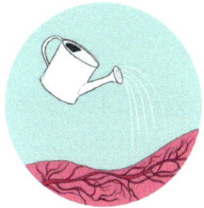

2. **Preparation for pregnancy:** Progesterone prepares the endometrium for possible implantation by encouraging the growth of blood vessels and glands within the uterine lining. This ensures that the embryo will have the necessary nutrients and support for early development

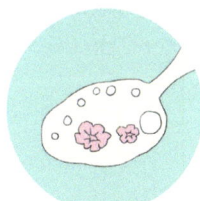

3. **Support during early pregnancy:** If fertilisation occurs, the corpus luteum secretes progesterone until the placenta takes over around the 8th to 10th week of pregnancy. Progesterone continues to support the uterine lining and help maintain the pregnancy

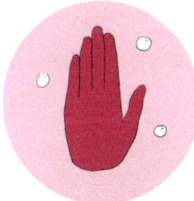

4. **Suppression of further ovulation:** Progesterone, in conjunction with high levels of oestrogen, helps prevent the release of additional eggs from the ovaries during the same menstrual cycle so you don't ovulate multiple times at random times in the cycle!

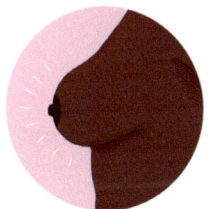

5. **Breast changes:** Progesterone, along with oestrogen, contributes to breast development and preparation for potential breastfeeding. It can also give you the breast tenderness you may notice in the run-up to your period

Progesterone levels change throughout the cycle

If pregnancy doesn't occur, the corpus luteum regresses, leading to a drop in progesterone levels. This decline triggers the shedding of the uterine lining, resulting in menstruation (aka your period).

The rise and fall of progesterone is important, because while it is important to have a thick endometrium for pregnancy to occur, it is also important for the thick lining to be shed. Otherwise, the lining can continue to thicken in response to oestrogen, and potentially could develop into endometrial cancer if left unchecked.

Even after the menopause, progesterone is still important for anyone who still has a uterus. If you opt for hormone replacement therapy (HRT) to help improve the symptoms of the perimenopause, the oestrogen component is important for helping to improve hot flushes, tiredness, and other effects.

However, if you do take HRT and you still have your uterus, it it is important to counter-balance the effect the oestrogen has on thickening the endometrium by adding in some progesterone. (More on this in Chapter 9 on the menopause!)

Other important hormones

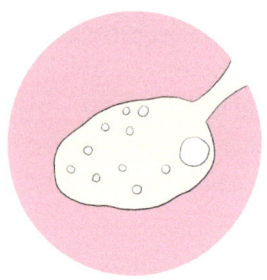 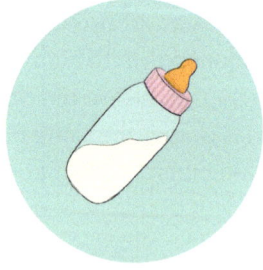 

FSH and LH:
the dynamic duo

Prolactin:
the milk maker

Oxytocin:
the love hormone

Follicle-stimulating hormone (FSH) and luteinising hormone (LH): the dynamic duo

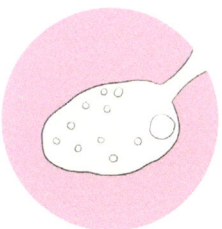

FSH and LH are hormones that are released by the pituitary gland, a small gland located at the base of the brain. They work together to regulate the menstrual cycle. FSH stimulates the growth of ovarian follicles, which house developing eggs. LH triggers ovulation, the release of a mature egg from the follicle, allowing it to potentially be fertilised.

If you notice your periods become irregular, testing these hormones is often one of the first things your doctor will do, because they are closely related to how often you ovulate.

Prolactin: the milk maker

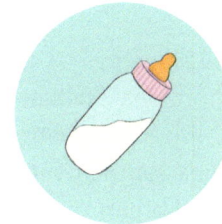

While not directly involved in the menstrual cycle, prolactin is worth mentioning for its role in lactation.

Prolactin is released by the pituitary gland, where its main role is stimulating milk production in the mammary glands after childbirth. High levels of prolactin can suppress ovulation, which is why you are less likely to fall pregnant while breastfeeding (although it's not impossible – see Chapter 6 on contraception for more on this!).

Oxytocin: the love hormone

Oxytocin, often called the 'love hormone' or 'bonding hormone', is primarily produced in a part of the brain known as the hypothalamus and is released by part of the pituitary gland.

One of its major roles occurs in pregnancy, as part of labour and childbirth. Surges of oxytocin levels stimulate contractions of the uterine muscles, facilitating the delivery of the baby.

This hormone also plays a pivotal role after birth, as it helps the uterus to contract and limits excessive bleeding after birth. It also plays an important role in breastfeeding, triggering the let-down reflex that allows milk to flow from the mammary glands. Additionally, oxytocin fosters maternal bonding and affectionate behaviours towards infants, promoting a strong emotional connection between mothers and their babies.

Beyond reproduction, oxytocin influences social interactions, intimacy, and stress regulation. It gets released after physical touch such as hugging someone and helps to strengthen emotional bonds and reduces stress by creating a sense of comfort and security.

During sex, oxytocin levels rise significantly, enhancing emotional intimacy and attachment between partners. This hormone not only deepens the emotional connection but also contributes to overall feelings of pleasure and satisfaction.

'Balancing' your hormones is a myth!

The idea that hormones need to be perfectly balanced at all times is a common misconception. In fact, it's more accurate to view hormonal fluctuations as a natural and dynamic part of the menstrual cycle. Misleading claims spread quickly on social media that if we choose certain foods, supplements, or lifestyle changes we could achieve a state of hormonal equilibrium.

In fact, our hormones are supposed to shift throughout the menstrual cycle, with various hormones like oestrogen and progesterone rising and falling in a coordinated dance. These fluctuations are essential for regulating processes such as ovulation, menstruation, and preparing the uterine lining for potential pregnancy.

In reality, attempting to 'balance' hormones constantly may not only be unattainable but also unnecessary for overall health and well-being. By dispelling the myth that there is a need for constant hormonal balance, we can promote a healthier understanding of the menstrual cycle and empower ourselves to embrace the natural variability of our hormonal health. This perspective encourages a more inclusive and accepting approach towards the diverse experiences that people have with their menstrual cycles. It also places less guilt on the shoulders of individuals, because it is not your 'fault' your symptoms are occurring. Rather than liberating us as modern women and people who menstruate, it actually suggests bodies are breaking down from the strain modern life places on individuals, and that our bodies need to accomplish more under ever-demanding social and economic conditions.

This term 'balance' to describe symptoms in relation to our hormones is ambiguous and can actually signify the very opposite of harmony and moderation. Instead, we should be tracking symptoms across the cycle, and seeking advice from medical professionals if they are problematic, so we can be given specific and relevant advice rather than buying into expensive self-help products.

MYTH 'We should adjust our working patterns, eating habits and exercise patterns based on our menstrual cycle'

FACT This is partly true. Many people do naturally adjust their working patterns, eating habits, and exercise routines in response to the different phases of their menstrual cycle. Hormonal fluctuations throughout the cycle can influence energy levels, mood, and physical performance, leading to changes in how women approach their daily activities. For instance, during the follicular phase, when oestrogen levels rise, you may experience increased energy and focus, making it an ideal time for high-intensity exercise, lifting heavier weights and increasing productivity. Conversely, during the luteal phase, higher progesterone levels may lead to fatigue and increased cravings, prompting a shift towards more rest and comfort foods.

Evidence suggests that exercise performance may be slightly lower during the early days of the menstrual cycle (the early follicular phase) compared to other times in the cycle.[1] However, the differences found between studies are quite large, which suggests that the results might depend on how the research was done, the characteristics of the women studied, and how performance was measured.

continued...

Because of this variation, the current evidence isn't strong enough to suggest specific advice on changing exercise routines based on the menstrual cycle. Instead, it's better to listen to your own body and adjust exercise based on how you feel during different phases of the cycle.

Also, while this might seem like sensible advice for optimising well-being, it may not be practical for everyone, especially those in demanding jobs like teaching or healthcare. These professions often require consistent performance regardless of where you are in your menstrual cycle, making it difficult to adjust work patterns or take additional rest when needed. For many people in these fields, understanding their menstrual cycle can still be helpful for self-care and planning around their more flexible activities, but it's not always possible to align their work schedules with their body's natural rhythms.

Conditions associated with differences in reproductive hormones

Polycystic ovary syndrome (PCOS)

PCOS is a common health condition that affects people with ovaries, typically during their reproductive years. It involves a difference in the balance of reproductive hormones, which leads to various symptoms and potential long-term health risks. The cause of PCOS is not yet known but it often runs in families. If any of your relatives (mother, aunts, sisters) are affected with PCOS, your risk of developing PCOS may be increased.

Polycystic ovaries are larger than normal ovaries and have twice the number of follicles, which are the precursor of eggs. It is important to note that not everyone with polycystic ovaries has PCOS. It is estimated that 30% of women and people with ovaries have polycystic ovaries,[2] but PCOS as a syndrome itself is less common, affecting around 10% depending on criteria applied.[3]

A diagnosis is made when you have any two of the following:

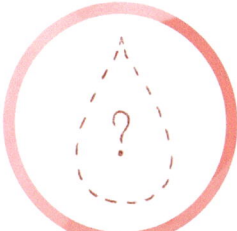

Irregular, infrequent periods or no periods at all

Higher levels of testosterone as shown by blood tests and/or increase in facial/ body hair

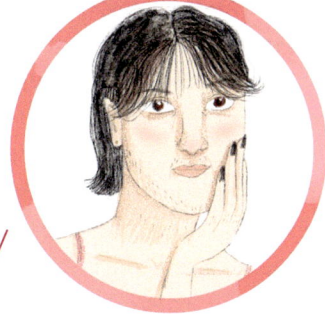

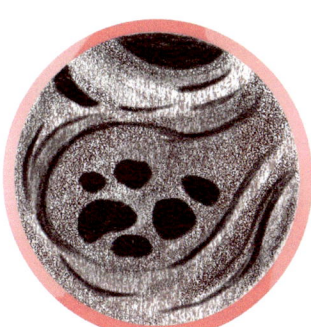

An ultrasound scan that shows polycystic ovaries

Other symptoms can include:

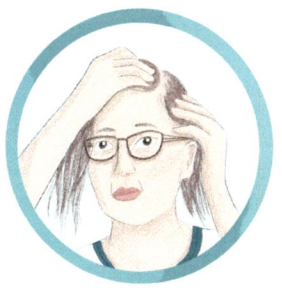

Being overweight or difficulty losing weight

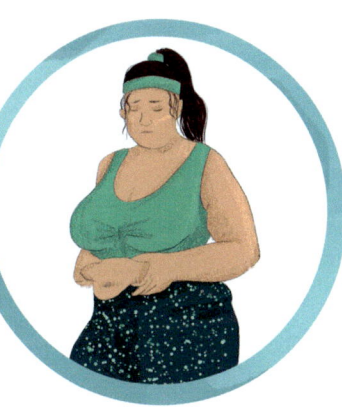

A loss of hair on head

Oily skin and acne

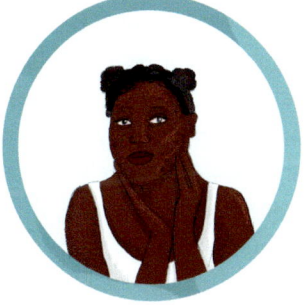

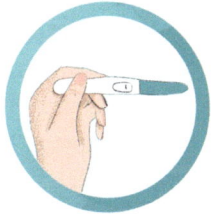

Difficulty falling pregnant

How is it diagnosed?

The range of symptoms in PCOS varies widely; some individuals experience few or no symptoms, while others may struggle with every symptom listed. For example, some people still have fairly regular periods but only notice occasional changes, while others may have no periods for months or even years. Weight gain and difficulty losing weight are common, but not universal, as is excessive hair growth, which can vary from light to more pronounced. Skin issues like acne and dark patches, along with fertility challenges and mood disturbances, also differ greatly, making PCOS a highly individualised condition that requires personalised management.

The symptoms that PCOS causes are related to changes in how your body manages certain hormones:

- **Raised androgens:** These are a family of hormones that includes testosterone. Androgens are produced in small amounts by the ovaries. People with PCOS have slightly higher than typical levels of androgens and this is associated with many of the symptoms of the condition

- **Insulin resistance:** Insulin is a hormone that controls the level of glucose (a type of sugar) in the blood. If you have PCOS, your body may not respond to insulin (this is known as insulin resistance), leading to a rise in glucose levels. To try to prevent high glucose, your body produces even more insulin.

  This excess insulin can stimulate the ovaries to produce more androgens (male hormones), which can lead to weight gain, irregular periods, fertility problems, and higher levels of testosterone. While insulin resistance in PCOS increases the risk of developing type 2 diabetes, having PCOS doesn't guarantee that diabetes will occur – it's one of many factors that contribute to the risk

- **Infrequent ovulation:** Polycystic ovaries contain many small follicles, which each contain an egg that has started to grow, but do not reach a mature size. This interferes with ovulation, as the egg does not get released and instead remains small. PCOS also results in raised levels of hormones such as LH, which further interferes with the messaging and can contribute to infrequent or absent menstrual cycles. People with PCOS who have infrequent ovulation may take longer to conceive and, without ovulation, other hormones such as progesterone can be affected

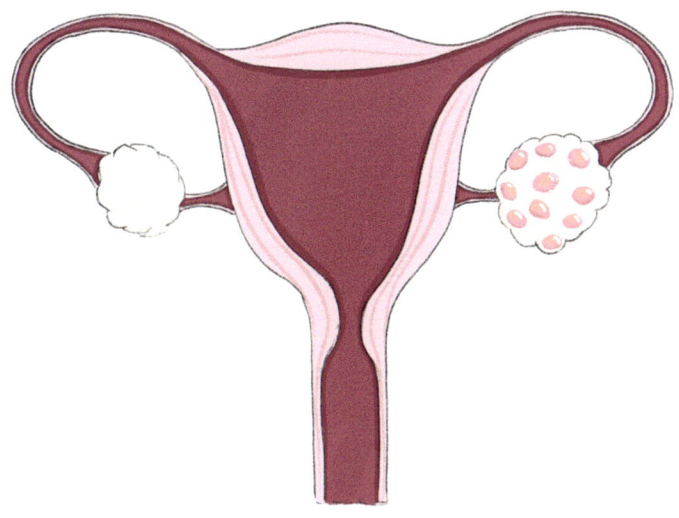

Can it be cured?

Currently, there is no single cure for PCOS, and medical treatments aim to manage and reduce the symptoms or consequences of having PCOS. Treatments are generally available to help manage specific symptoms, like irregular periods or acne. However, we are moving towards taking a more holistic approach, considering your overall well-being and priorities to help determine which treatments are right for you at different times in your life.

For managing PCOS, adopting a healthy lifestyle and focusing on weight management are recommended as the first steps, as they can be just as effective as medication alone for certain PCOS symptoms!

This includes making changes to your diet and exercise routine, with the goal of preventing weight gain; achieving a modest weight loss if needed, or maintaining a healthy weight. For those above the healthy weight range, losing 5–10% of body weight can make a big difference.[4] In fact, just that change alone without any extra medication can be enough to restart regular ovulation, and create a more predictable pattern to your periods. A balanced diet is recommended, as no specific diet has proven to be better for PCOS.

For exercise, aim for at least 150 minutes of moderate activity or 75 minutes of vigorous activity per week for general health, and more if weight loss is a goal. Including muscle-strengthening exercises twice a week is also beneficial. Setting specific, measurable, and realistic goals can help with sticking to these changes. Like giving yourself targets to motivate you, such as 'couch to 5k' or a goal of running a half-marathon. You don't have to do it alone, so speak to a trainer, physiotherapist or health professional if you need specific support. Improving lifestyle and weight management can positively impact various aspects of PCOS, making periods more regular but, more importantly, benefitting your overall health.

Options for the medical treatments depend on which symptom bothers you the most. This means that if it's the hair growth, certain types of the combined contraceptive pill or laser for hair removal can be effective. If your main concern is acne, again certain contraceptive pills or creams can be used.

The combined pill can be used to help regulate periods if never knowing when your period will come is frustrating and you prefer to be able to predict when you will have a bleed. If you go long periods of time (more than 3 months) without a period, then hormonal pills may be recommended to keep the lining of the womb thin and protect against endometrial cancer.

PCOS can affect fertility by making it harder to ovulate, which is necessary to conceive a pregnancy spontaneously. To help with this, ovulation induction medications like letrozole and clomifene citrate are often used as the first step to stimulate ovulation. These treatments are effective and generally safe, but it is also important to be aware of the risks such as ovarian hyperstimulation syndrome (OHSS) and an increased chance of multiple pregnancies, requiring close monitoring by a healthcare provider. If these approaches are unsuccessful, assisted reproductive technologies like in vitro fertilisation (IVF) may be considered.

What does it mean long term?

While PCOS cannot be cured, it is a condition that can be effectively managed with the right treatment strategies. Being aware of the longer-term risks allows us to put in place methods to reduce or eliminate the complications. While PCOS may increase the likelihood of challenges such as insulin resistance or type 2 diabetes and cardiovascular issues, taking steps to adopt a healthy lifestyle can reduce these risks.

People with PCOS can be at a higher risk of developing endometrial cancer because they often experience irregular periods or no periods at all (known as oligo-ovulation and anovulation). These conditions mean that the lining of the uterus (endometrium) is exposed to oestrogen without the balancing effect of progesterone, which can lead to an overgrowth of the lining (endometrial hyperplasia) and, over time, increase the risk of cancer.

To reduce this risk, it's important for individuals with PCOS to have a menstrual bleed at least every 3 months. This helps to shed the thickened uterine lining and lowers the chance of it developing into cancer. If someone is not trying to get pregnant, taking hormonal medications like the combined oral contraceptive pill is often recommended to regulate bleeds and keep the endometrium thin. These pills not only help to make bleeding more predictable but also manage other symptoms of PCOS, like excess androgen levels.

PMS and PMDD

Premenstrual syndrome (PMS) refers to a combination of physical, emotional, and behavioural symptoms that tend to occur in the days or weeks leading up to a menstrual period.

What causes PMS?

PMS is caused by hormonal fluctuations that particularly occur during the second half of the menstrual cycle. After ovulation, levels of progesterone rise to prepare the body for a potential pregnancy, while oestrogen levels fluctuate. If pregnancy does not occur, both hormone levels drop sharply, triggering PMS symptoms in some individuals. These hormonal changes can affect brain chemicals such as serotonin, which influences mood and emotional regulation, potentially leading to symptoms like irritability, sadness, and anxiety.

The exact cause of PMS is not fully understood, and we don't really know why it affects some people more than others, but it is thought to involve a heightened sensitivity to hormonal changes. Other factors, such as stress, poor sleep, or an unhealthy diet, may exacerbate symptoms. While PMS can be challenging, lifestyle adjustments, stress management, and, in some cases, medical interventions can help manage symptoms effectively.

The pill is a treatment for PMS because it helps stabilise hormone levels, preventing the sharp fluctuations in oestrogen and progesterone that can trigger PMS symptoms, which aims to lead to more consistent moods and fewer physical symptoms like breast tenderness.

What are the symptoms?

From bloating and headaches to bad skin and sensitive moods, up to 90% of us will experience at least one PMS symptom before our period.[5] Not everyone experiences all PMS symptoms, but some of the most common are:

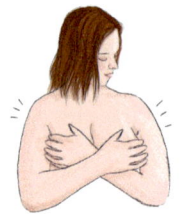

- **Physical symptoms:** These can include bloating, breast tenderness, headaches, fatigue, and changes in appetite

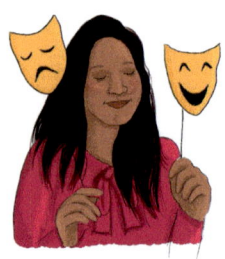

- **Withdrawing and detachment:** Social gatherings and parties can suddenly seem less than appealing and your motivation is at a monthly low

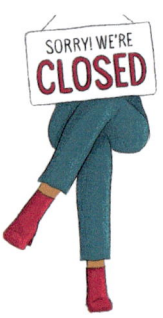

- **Low sex drive:** Oestrogen takes a nosedive in this part of the cycle and takes libido as well as vaginal lubrication along with it

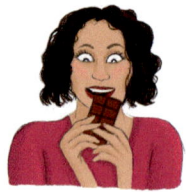

- **Change in appetite:** You could be craving more of certain foods around this time or your appetite could disappear. It's common to feel like eating sweet, carb-heavy 'comfort food'

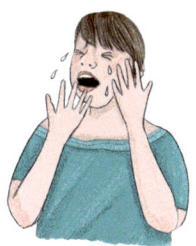

- **Feeling anxious, irritable, or sensitive:** You might find yourself getting teary, feeling extra stressed, or insecure

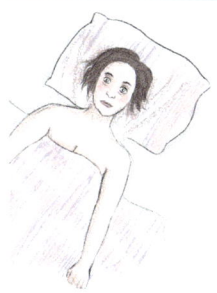

- **Feeling tired:** Despite feeling fatigued and lethargic, you might find it hard to fall asleep at night

It's important to remember that PMS affects people differently, and not everyone experiences all of these symptoms. Also, the severity and duration of symptoms can vary from person to person.

Sometimes, the symptoms of PMS can go beyond just bothersome, manifesting as premenstrual dysphoric disorder (PMDD) – a severe form of PMS. This can mean that in the run-up to your period, hormones can also amplify feelings like anxiety, depression, and other mental health conditions that someone may already experience.

PMDD

Around 20–40% of women experience moderate to severe premenstrual symptoms (PMS).[6] However, between 2% and 6% of women experience symptoms that prevent them from functioning in normal daily life.[7] This is premenstrual dysphoric disorder (PMDD).

What is PMDD, and how does it differ from PMS?

PMDD is characterised by intense physical and emotional symptoms that significantly disrupt daily life. Like PMS, PMDD is linked to hormonal changes during the luteal phase of the menstrual cycle, but the emotional and psychological symptoms in PMDD are far more severe. While PMS may cause mood swings and discomfort, PMDD symptoms include debilitating depression, anxiety, irritability, and even feelings of hopelessness, which resemble major depressive or anxiety disorders. However, PMDD is unique in that these symptoms are directly tied to the menstrual cycle and typically subside a few days after menstruation begins.

The impact and outlook of PMDD

PMDD can profoundly impact a person's life, affecting relationships, work, and overall well-being. The extreme emotional symptoms can make it difficult to perform daily activities, and the recurring nature of the condition can be exhausting and isolating. Treatment for PMDD often involves a combination of approaches: lifestyle changes such as regular exercise and a healthy diet may help, while medications like selective serotonin reuptake inhibitors (SSRIs) can be effective. Hormonal treatments, such as oral contraceptives, can also help regulate the hormonal fluctuations that trigger symptoms. For those struggling with PMDD, professional support and personalised care are essential to manage the condition and improve quality of life.

Coping with PMS

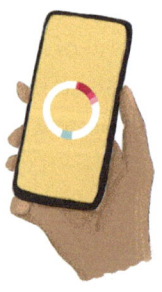

Tracking your cycle is usually the first step towards managing the impact of the symptoms of PMS, so you know what is coming and when. You might find it helpful to make little adjustments to your schedule if you find certain days particularly challenging.

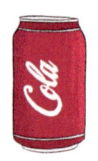

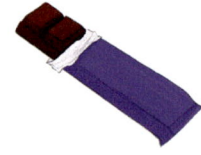

Following a balanced diet, without too much sugar, but also without excessive restrictions may keep energy levels more consistent, and getting enough sleep can help. Regular exercise is beneficial to improve PMS symptoms (even if it is the last thing you feel like doing), especially aerobic exercise, such as walking, jogging, or skipping. Even just switching up your route to work to incorporate 30 minutes walking each day could make a noticeable difference. Some people find relaxation techniques like deep breathing or yoga to be beneficial.

Studies have shown that smoking can make PMS symptoms worse, which is another pretty good reason to stop![8]

PMS can affect our body clocks, making it more difficult to sleep even if we're feeling lethargic. To try and counter this, try putting your phone away before bedtime because the bright light before bed can make it harder to fall asleep. Instead, dim the lights and do something you find relaxing like nestling down with a good book before shutting your eyes for the night. Ensure the room you're sleeping in is ventilated; opening the window for a short period of time each day can help to increase oxygen levels in the room.

Stress has a habit of making any symptom worse, including those of PMS. Some people find that massage, mindfulness, and meditation really help. Also plan your events carefully if you need to; don't feel guilty about saying 'no' to social occasions! If you struggle with concentration and fatigue, it might be helpful to try and avoid taking any big or important decisions around this time.

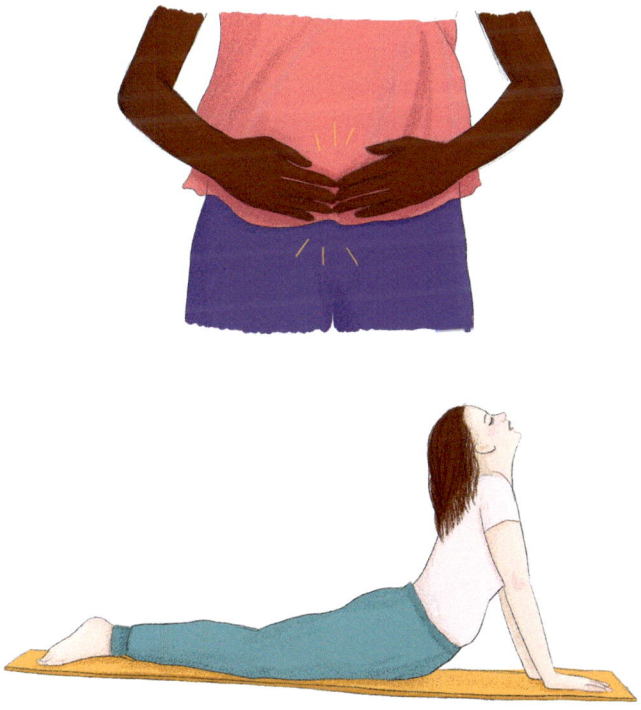

Treatment options

If your PMS is having a big impact on your life, you do not just have to accept it as something you need to put up with. As well as some lifestyle changes explained above, there are some other options:

- **Psychological treatments:** The mood changes of PMS can be a challenge, and cognitive behavioural therapy (CBT) has been shown to be effective. It can help you learn new ways of managing some of your symptoms to reduce their impact on your daily life

- **Complementary treatments:** If you aren't keen to take hormones, UK guidelines suggest supplements of calcium, vitamin D, Vitex agnus-castus (a herb known as chasteberry) or Ginkgo biloba may be helpful. Evening primrose oil can reduce breast tenderness.[9] However, it is important to note that the evidence supporting their use is limited

- **Hormonal medications:** An effective way to control the symptoms of PMS is to take the combined contraceptive pill (particularly those containing the hormone drospirenone such as Yasmin); these have been shown to be really helpful. To keep hormone levels steady, you can take this pill continuously rather than with a break. (Check out Chapter 6 on contraception for more!)

- **Non-hormonal medications:** These include antidepressant medications such as SSRIs, which may be helpful for the mood-related PMS symptoms. These can be taken on a daily basis for 2 weeks before your period, or all the way through your cycle

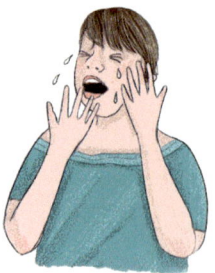 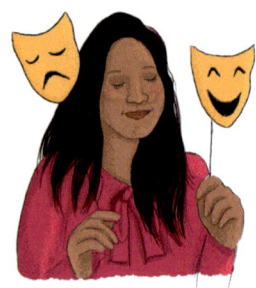

If the above options are not effective enough, your doctor can adjust the doses of medication or consider the next-step hormonal option such as gonadotropin-releasing hormone (GnRH) analogue injections. These cause a temporary and reversible menopause, so it prevents ovulation, meaning you will not have any periods. This option is also helpful to confirm the diagnosis as we can determine if taking away your menstrual cycles resolves all of your symptoms, meaning that you have true PMS or PMDD.

Surgical options for managing PMS are typically considered as a last resort for severe symptoms where other treatments have not been effective. The main surgical option is a hysterectomy, which involves the removal of the uterus, often combined with the removal of the ovaries (oophorectomy). This surgery stops the menstrual cycle and, therefore, the hormonal fluctuations that cause PMS. By removing the potential for ovulation, it therefore makes you immediately menopausal. This means the surgical option to treat PMS symptoms should only be considered in someone who has completed their family or does not wish to fall pregnant in the future. Such extensive surgery has benefits, and also disadvantages, so should be discussed at length with your own doctor.

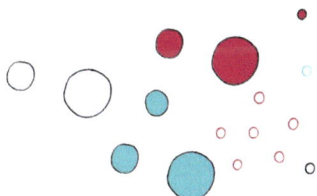

Hormones are vital for driving the menstrual cycle, orchestrating processes like ovulation, preparing the uterine lining for potential pregnancy, and triggering menstruation when pregnancy doesn't occur. Their interaction ensures the cycle runs effectively. However, various factors such as PCOS, thyroid disorders, or stress can influence how hormones function, affecting cycle regularity and overall reproductive health. Recognising their importance helps us understand key aspects of menstrual health and address potential concerns effectively.

What it can feel like to go through fertility treatment

UNLUCKY

ROLLERCOASTER OF EMOTIONS

OVERWHELMING

TIME PRESSURE

SO MANY NEEDLES

NEVER-ENDING

COSTLY

POSTCODE LOTTERY

EXHAUSTING

PAPERWORK

JUGGLING WORK AND TREATMENTS

FEELING HOPEFUL

ALIENATED FROM THE SUPPORTING PARTNER

CHAPTER 5

Fertility:
getting pregnant

Fertility, the ability to conceive and create a new life, requires a complex interplay of different factors. While it may seem that for some this process is really easy (they don't even have to think about falling pregnant and it just happens), the reality is that a huge number of individual processes need to line up perfectly to reach the final outcome of giving birth to a live baby.

How your fertility works

The female reproductive system revolves around the menstrual cycle, a roughly 28-day rhythm orchestrated by hormones. It begins with the release of an egg from one of the ovaries, a process known as ovulation. This egg, poised for potential fertilisation, journeys down the fallopian tube in the hope of meeting some sperm. Meanwhile, the uterus prepares a nurturing environment, thickening its lining in anticipation of a fertilised egg.

If that fertilised egg arrives close to the womb, it needs to be able to successfully implant into the lining of the womb (the endometrium) where it can begin to divide and enlarge, developing into an embryo, then a fetus, and eventually into a baby.

If you want to understand more about the menstrual cycle, check out Chapter 2 and 4!

How long does it take to get pregnant?

Statistics suggest that around 50% of all pregnancies are unplanned, and we all know people who never consciously worried about when and how they might get pregnant, as they fell pregnant without even trying.[1] However, for many of us, trying for a baby can be an overwhelming time, with the process taking over every inch of our existence.

When you feel desperate to see a positive pregnancy test, and it comes back negative each month, it can leave you wondering how long is 'normal' for the process to take, and how long you should keep waiting?

How long should I keep trying for?

The time it takes to get pregnant can vary for each couple, with a lot of factors coming into play. The majority of people (over 90%) having regular unprotected sexual intercourse will get pregnant within a year and around one in three people will get pregnant within a month of trying.[2] However, it's important to remember these are just statistics to help guide your expectations and there are no hard and fast rules.

This is why, generally, doctors advise testing for fertility issues only after a couple has been trying for over a year to conceive while having regular intercourse. There are certain caveats to this though, because there is no point in waiting a whole year if either partner already knows that they have an underlying issue which may affect their fertility, such as a blocked fallopian tube, or a known testicular problem.

What does regular sex mean?

When you hear people talk about regular sex, they mean having unprotected ('penis-in-vagina') sex every 2 to 3 days throughout the month. It's normal for the pressure of needing to make time for sex regularly to feel stressful, especially if trying for a baby is taking longer than you expected.

While having sex every 2–3 days is optimal, this is not always possible for everyone. For example, not all couples are living together when trying for a baby, or they may have busy lives! Differing libido and desire levels can also make sex feel more like a chore, which becomes something you may dread.

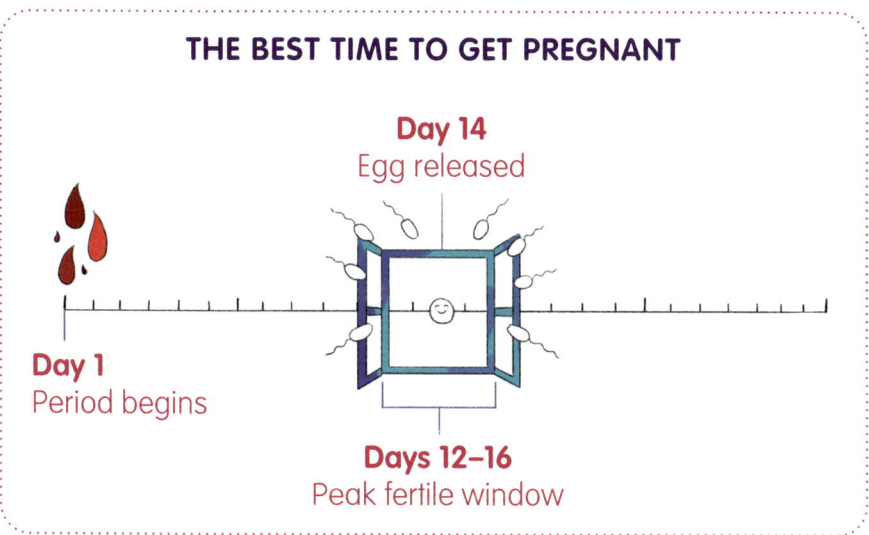

THE BEST TIME TO GET PREGNANT

Day 14
Egg released

Day 1
Period begins

Days 12–16
Peak fertile window

If you need to focus your efforts when you're trying for a baby, then the best time to have sex is around the specific days when an egg is released from your ovary, called ovulation. This usually occurs around day 14 of your cycle; 2 weeks after the first day of your period. The days before and the day after ovulation are the most fertile and this is sometimes called your 'fertile window'.

It can be helpful to track your periods in an app or use an ovulation calculator to try and tell you when your fertile window is. Then you can optimise the timing of intercourse, focusing your efforts, if you need to, around the 5-day fertile window leading up to and just after ovulation occurs. Even if you aren't trying to conceive just yet, it can be helpful to track at least three menstrual cycles so that you know what to expect when you do get going, although the longer you can track your cycles for, the better you will be able to get to know your fertile window and the signs your body gives you to indicate ovulation, and when your period is coming. (More about cycle tracking in Chapter 2 on periods!)

> **Myth** 'You need to have sex every day to increase your chances of falling pregnant'
>
> **Fact** Actually, having sex too frequently could decrease sperm number and quality and is unlikely to improve your chances of falling pregnant. So, every other day during the fertile window is fine!

What factors influence your fertility?

Fertility is influenced by many factors, and sometimes challenges can arise from one or both partners, or the cause may remain unknown.[3] Approximately 30% of fertility issues are linked to problems affecting the female partner, or those with a uterus and ovaries, while another 30% are related to issues affecting the male partner, or those with testes. The remaining 30–40% of fertility problems either involve factors from both partners or have no identifiable cause.

The following are associated with reduced fertility:

- **Smoking:** If you smoke it is likely to take you longer to get pregnant than a non-smoker, with the chances cut by almost half every month. Smoking also negatively affects semen by reducing sperm count, motility, and also increases the risk of DNA damage in sperm leading to fertility issues and a higher likelihood of genetic abnormalities. If either partner smokes, the best thing you can do before getting pregnant is stop smoking

- **Alcohol:** Drinking alcohol is linked to fertility problems. If you drink a lot and often, you may find it more difficult to get pregnant. Heavy drinking can also contribute to heavy, irregular, or absent periods. This means you are less likely to be ovulating regularly. Like smoking, drinking alcohol can also reduce sperm count, motility, and overall quality. If you are planning a pregnancy, it is advisable for both partners to minimise their alcohol intake during this time

- **Sexually transmitted infections:** Chlamydia and gonorrhoea are two of the most common sexually transmitted infections. Many people with chlamydia and gonorrhoea don't have any symptoms at all. Both can lead to reduced fertility in either partner if they are not treated. If you think you or your partner might be at risk of a sexually transmitted infection, it's important to go for a check-up at a sexual health clinic before you start trying to conceive

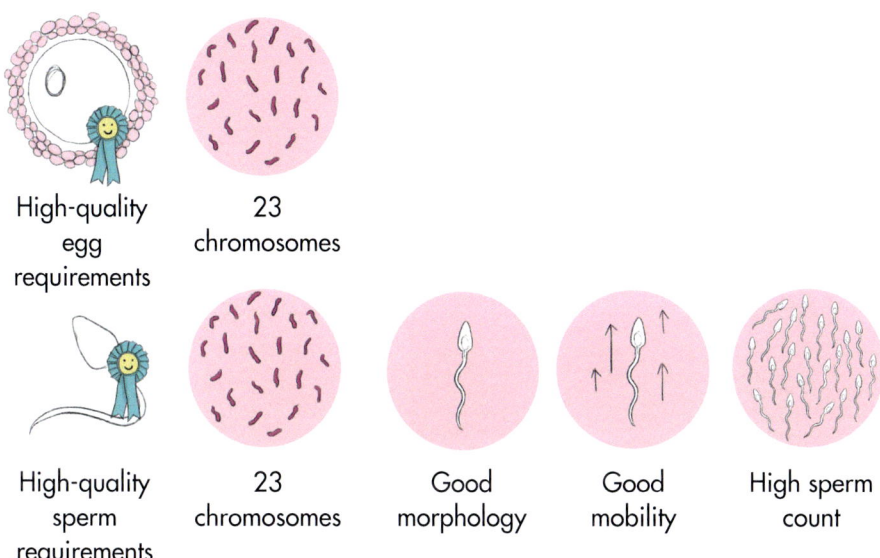

High-quality egg requirements

23 chromosomes

High-quality sperm requirements

23 chromosomes

Good morphology

Good mobility

High sperm count

Age and getting pregnant

It is hard enough trying to have a successful career, fighting through the challenges of ever-increasing costs of living, not to mention finding someone that you actually want to start a family with, so it is incredibly frustrating to be frequently reminded about the ticking biological clock!

As a gynaecologist I feel constantly torn – I want to tell you that modern technology is amazing, that you can achieve anything and shouldn't be held back by being someone with ovaries. But at the same time, I feel compelled to tell you that no matter how good our technology is getting, the facts haven't really changed that much.

The single biggest factor that affects our fertility is age.

Even if you go through in vitro fertilisation (IVF), it still remains true that IVF is more successful the younger you are when the process starts.

This shouldn't be scary information – nobody should feel pressured to have a baby when they aren't ready. Instead, it should be empowering – knowing this fact means that, when you are ready, by acting sooner rather than delaying the decision, you will have better chances of falling pregnant, and that has to be a good thing!

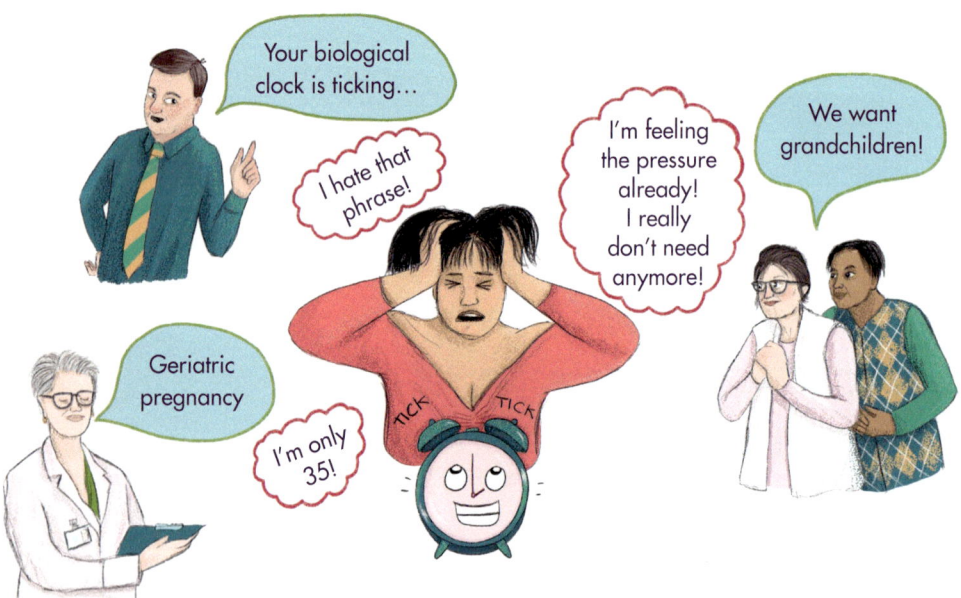

Why does age matter?

It can be intimidating to be told that a pregnancy after the age of 35 puts you in the 'advanced maternal age' category or, even worse still, you may hear the term 'geriatric pregnancy', which is a phrase that should be completely banished! Either way, remember that pregnancy after you are 35 is still very common and has excellent outcomes.

The 'biological clock' that you may have heard of refers to the limited time during which the ovaries can produce high-quality eggs regularly enough to conceive a pregnancy. The time starts when you get your first period and ends when you enter the menopause. It may come as a surprise that your peak reproductive years are actually between your late teens and late 20s.

As you get older, it can take longer to become pregnant and the likelihood that you may need to access medical help with getting pregnant increases. This is because the eggs in your ovaries are also getting older, causing a reduction in your fertility. You are born with a finite number of eggs. Over time, this number, along with the quality of the eggs, decreases because we tend to release the best eggs earlier, so as we get older the ones left behind tend to be of lower quality.

Fertility will usually start to decline rapidly 5–10 years before the menopause, as you begin to run out of good-quality eggs for ovulation. The majority of women experience menopause between the ages of 45 and 55. When your body goes through the menopause it is influenced by a lot of different factors including your family history, when your first period started, and the number of times you have been pregnant. (More on this in Chapter 9 on the menopause!)

These statistics can be scary, especially if this is your reality. It's important to remember that although fertility does change as you age, the changes are gradual – pregnancy doesn't become impossible overnight!

For couples having regular unprotected sex:[4]

- Around 7 out of 10 women aged 30 will conceive within 1 year

- Around 6 out of 10 women aged 35 will conceive within 1 year

- Around 4 out of 10 women aged 40 will conceive within 1 year

Age and male fertility

Male fertility also declines with age, although the decline is slower in comparison to females. Over the age of 40, there is a gradual decrease in sperm quality, including lower sperm count, reduced motility, and an increase in DNA damage. Additionally, older age in males is associated with a higher risk of genetic mutations in sperm, which can impact the chances of successful conception and increase the risk of certain genetic disorders in offspring.

What if you aren't ready to try for a pregnancy just yet?

Knowing that age has a significant impact on your fertility means that you can explore your options. While ideally you would start trying to conceive earlier than later, this isn't always possible. One option to consider is whether you should freeze your eggs.

Modern medicine has made some truly remarkable leaps in recent years, many of which are required to keep pace with our changing society. There are many reasons women may look into freezing their eggs, and these may include:

- Those facing infertility for medical reasons, such as chemotherapy for cancers

- Social reasons such as not having met the right partner and wishing to delay pregnancy until later life

Egg freezing is a procedure to preserve eggs by extracting them from the ovaries, and freezing and storing them for later use. In the future you may choose to have the eggs thawed, fertilised via IVF, and transferred to the uterus as an embryo to enable a pregnancy. When done for social reasons, it can be argued that this process extends the window of opportunity for single women and people with a uterus to find the right partner, and offers hope when fertility declines with age.

However, it is important to note that the procedure can be very expensive. As well as needing to cover the egg stimulation and harvesting, there is also the cost of storage and future fertility treatment. And, of course, there is no guarantee of success because even if you use those eggs for IVF later, they may not result in a successful pregnancy. Evidence suggests the best time to freeze eggs is before the age of 35 because the younger the person is when the eggs are frozen, the more eggs are likely to be retrieved, and the better quality they will be.[5]

When should you stop contraception?

All forms of contraception apart from sterilisation procedures are reversible, meaning they do not cause any lasting damage to your fertility. However, some types of contraception can cause a delay in getting pregnant after you stop taking it. For example, once you stop taking the progesterone-only injection for contraception there may be delay to your periods returning, meaning your underlying fertility may not return to your baseline for up to 1 year after the last injection.

The best time to stop hormonal contraception before trying to conceive depends on the type of contraception being used and how quickly its

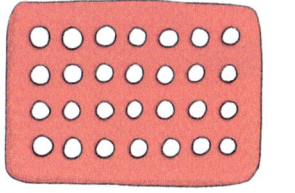 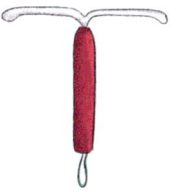 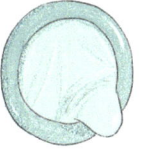 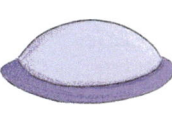

effects wear off. For most methods, such as the birth control pill, patch, or vaginal ring, ovulation will begin again within a few weeks to months after discontinuation, meaning it is possible to fall pregnant immediately. However, it may take up to 6 months for menstruation to become regular again.

For long-acting methods like the contraceptive injection (Depo-Provera), it may take longer, typically 6–12 months, for fertility to return to underlying levels. It's usually recommended to stop these methods earlier if planning to conceive soon. Intrauterine devices (IUDs) or implants can lead to immediate return of fertility once removed.

When you stop any form of contraception, some people may naturally fall pregnant immediately and for others it will take the full amount of time for the effects to wear off. There is no right time to stop contraception in advance of trying to conceive, but if you wish to allow your cycles to regulate and observe them for a few months before trying to conceive, you may prefer to stop hormonal contraception for 6 months before you are ready to fall pregnant. In that time, you may prefer to use barrier methods of contraception until you are ready to conceive. Check in with your doctor to discuss your plans for conceiving to come up with the right approach for you.

After stopping hormonal contraception, several changes may occur as your body adjusts to the removal of the external hormones. Most people will notice the return of their menstrual periods within a few weeks to a few months, although these may be irregular initially as hormone levels settle back into a regular pattern. Symptoms like cramping, mood swings, acne, or changes in libido, which were previously managed by contraception, might reappear as you return to your underlying hormone levels. These symptoms might flare initially but ease off over the next few months.

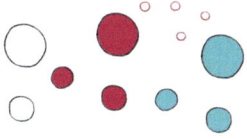

TOP TIPS FOR TRYING TO GET PREGNANT:

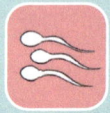 **HAVE REGULAR SEX:** Have sex every 2–3 days, focusing particularly around the time you are ovulating

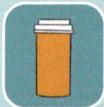 **TAKE FOLIC ACID DAILY:** Take folic acid every day – ideally you should aim to start taking folic acid supplements for 3 months before you start trying to conceive to ensure your levels build up

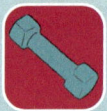 **FOCUS ON A HEALTHY LIFESTYLE:** Try to maintain a healthy weight and do regular exercise

 **AVOID ALCOHOL:** Cut down or stop drinking alcohol

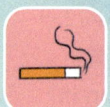 **STOP SMOKING**

When conceiving takes longer than expected ... aka subfertility

Subfertility is the term used to describe reduced levels of fertility, where it takes longer to fall pregnant than typically expected. Unlike infertility, where conception is not possible without medical intervention, subfertility means that pregnancy is still possible, but it may take longer – typically more than 12 months of regular, unprotected intercourse.

Subfertility can result from factors affecting either partner, including hormonal imbalances, issues with ovulation, low sperm quality, or anatomical problems in the reproductive system. It is often treatable with lifestyle changes, medications, or assisted reproductive technologies like IVF.

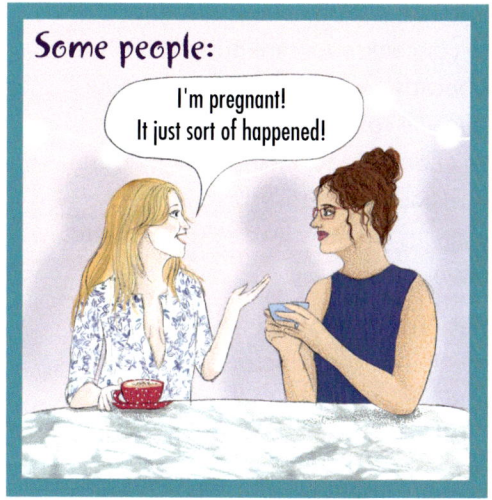

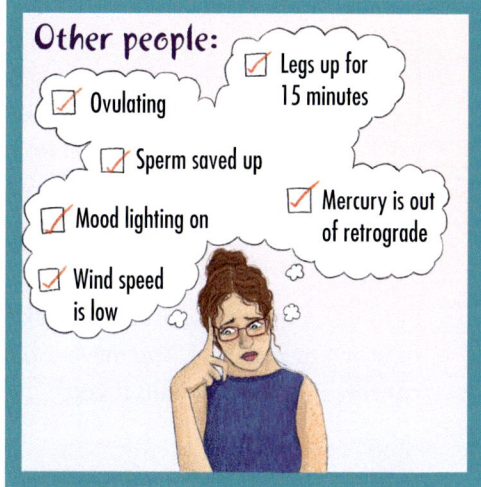

When should I get help with trying to get pregnant?

Around one in six couples will have difficulties getting pregnant.[6] If you are worried about how long it is taking, you can talk to your GP about your concerns, and they can discuss your lifestyle, general health, and medical history. They can run some initial investigations and give you advice on improving your chances of getting pregnant.

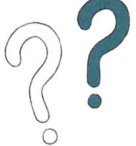

Many doctors will usually suggest waiting until at least a year of having regular sex without contraception before referring you for fertility tests. You should see your doctor after 12 months if you:

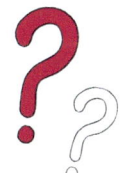

Are under 36

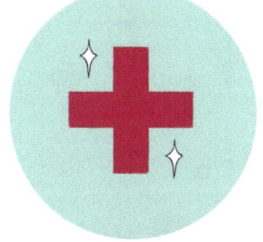

Have no medical problems

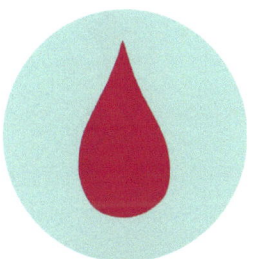

Have regular cycles

In many cases, even with a condition like severe endometriosis that affects fertility, it's often recommended to try to conceive spontaneously at first before pursuing fertility treatments. This is because even though doctors may be pessimistic and tell you it is unlikely you will conceive, it can actually be very difficult to predict who will and won't conceive spontaneously if given the opportunity. Regular intercourse while tracking your cycle to identify your fertile window can optimise your chances and may lead to spontaneous conception without immediate intervention.

In some cases, it's important to seek fertility advice sooner than 12 months of trying to conceive. You may wish to speak with your doctor if you don't conceive within 6 months if you:

 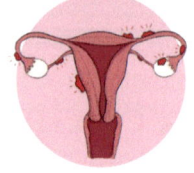 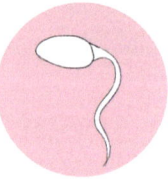 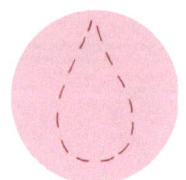

Are over 36   **Have a known fertility issue, such as endometriosis**   **Your partner has a known fertility issue**   **You are having no/irregular periods**

If you have significant concerns about your or your partner's fertility already, or if you are taking any medication which may have an effect on pregnancy, then see your doctor as soon as you plan to start trying to conceive.

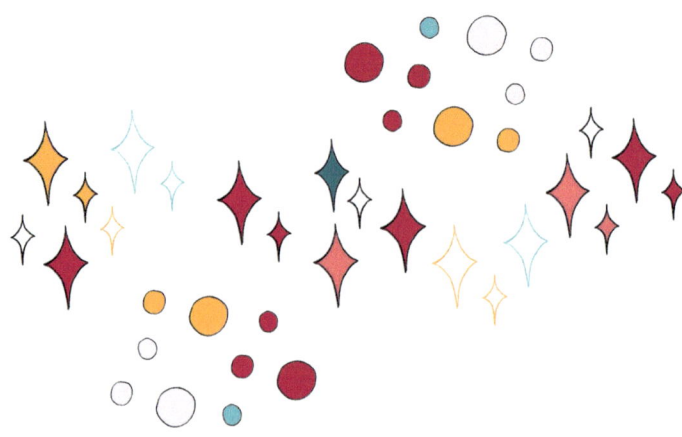

124

Causes of subfertility for females, or people with a womb and ovaries

In many cases of subfertility, no specific cause is found, but there are several key factors that can affect fertility in people with a womb and ovaries:

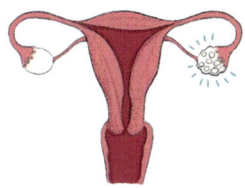

- **Ovulatory problems:** Ovulation, the release of an egg from the ovary, is essential for pregnancy. Conditions like PCOS or ageing can affect ovulation, egg quality, or both, leading to irregular or absent periods and difficulty conceiving

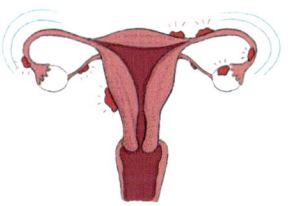

- **Blocked fallopian tubes:** The fallopian tubes provide the pathway for an egg to travel from the ovary to the uterus. Blockages caused by infections or conditions like endometriosis can prevent fertilisation or lead to complications like ectopic pregnancy

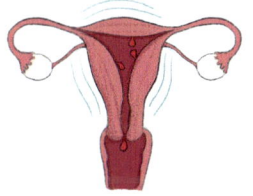

- **Uterine issues:** Structural problems in the uterus, such as fibroids or polyps, can make it harder for a fertilised egg to implant, potentially contributing to infertility or recurrent miscarriage

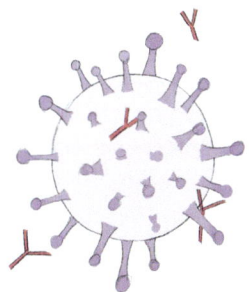

- **Autoimmune disorders:** Conditions like thyroid disease, lupus, or rheumatoid arthritis can disrupt the release of hormones, cause inflammation, or interfere with implantation and pregnancy, increasing the risk of fertility challenges or miscarriage. Proper medical management can improve outcomes

These factors highlight the complexity of fertility issues and the importance of individualising how we approach someone who is taking longer to conceive than expected.

How does male fertility work?

3. From there, during sexual arousal, the sperm travel through the **vas deferens**, a long tube that connects the epididymis to the urethra

4. As they move, fluids from the seminal vesicles and prostate are added, forming semen

5. Finally, the grand crescendo occurs during **ejaculation**, the semen is propelled through the **urethra** into the female reproductive tract

1. Male fertility centres around the production, maturation, and delivery of sperm. Sperm cells, created in the testes, undergo a process of development known as spermatogenesis

2. Once mature, the journey of sperm begins in the **testes**, where they are produced through a process called **spermatogenesis**. Once formed, they move into the **epididymis**, where they mature and gain the ability to swim

Causes of subfertility for males, or people with testes

Several factors and steps in the male reproductive system can contribute to fertility issues when disrupted:

- **Sperm production and transport issues:** Conditions such as testicular trauma, infections, or genetic factors can impair the production of healthy sperm in the testes. Blockages, swelling, or infections can prevent the normal transport of sperm, leading to infertility even with normal sperm production

- **Erectile dysfunction:** Difficulty achieving or maintaining an erection can hinder the ability to ejaculate and deliver sperm for fertilisation

- **Hormonal imbalances:** Imbalances in hormones such as testosterone, follicle-stimulating hormone (FSH), and luteinising hormone (LH) can affect sperm production and function

- **Retrograde ejaculation:** In retrograde ejaculation, semen is directed backward into the bladder instead of being expelled through the penis. This means those sperm don't make it to where they need to go!

- **Environmental and lifestyle factors:** Excessive heat around the testes, smoking, or excessive alcohol consumption can negatively impact sperm quality, count, and overall sperm health

Consulting with a healthcare provider or a fertility specialist can help identify the specific factors contributing to fertility issues and guide the development of a personalised treatment plan.

Investigating fertility – what tests may be offered?

If you have been trying to conceive without success, the next steps will usu-ally involve a range of tests, depending on individual circumstances, to see if there is a specific treatable cause that could explain the subfertility. Common investigations include blood tests, ultrasound scans, and tests to evaluate whether the fallopian tubes are open. For male partners, semen analysis is used to assess sperm count and quality. Not everyone will undergo all these tests; the investigations are tailored to the person's medical history and specific concerns. A health professional will guide you through which tests are most relevant based on individual needs.

Ultrasound scans

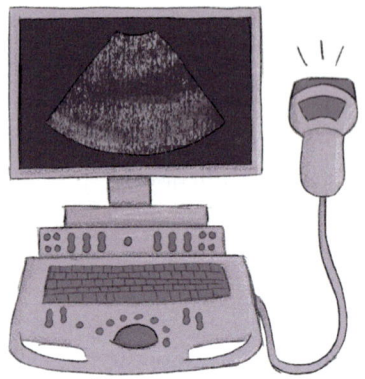

A transvaginal ultrasound scan will usually be carried out to look at your ovaries, womb, and fallopian tubes. This will involve a probe being inserted into the vagina to gain the best views of the reproductive organs.

The scan can give an initial indication of any issues that could affect fertility, such as endometriosis, fibroids, or cysts. These ultrasound scans can be a bit uncomfortable, but they shouldn't be painful. If you have vaginismus or struggle with smear tests, then talk to your doctor about what could make the process easier for you. This might include options such as inserting the probe yourself, having relaxing music playing in your headphones, or just having a longer appointment time.

Blood tests

Hormones are chemical messengers that regulate the reproductive system, enabling ovulation and implantation of an embryo. If hormonal issues are suspected as a cause of difficulty conceiving, your doctor may request blood tests to check levels of hormones like LH, FSH, oestrogen, progesterone, thyroid hormones, and testosterone. These hormones fluctuate throughout the menstrual cycle, so you may need to go back for specific blood tests on certain days of your cycle.

Ovarian reserve tests

Ovarian reserve tests can be used to assess the number and quality of eggs remaining in the ovaries, helping doctors evaluate fertility potential and predict how someone might respond to different types of treatment.

Ovarian reserve (aka how many eggs remain in the ovaries) can be assessed by measuring two important hormones in your blood:

- Follicle-stimulating hormone (FSH)
- Anti-Müllerian hormone (AMH)

Another way to assess the ovarian reserve is by ultrasound. During a scan, the follicles in the ovaries are counted to give a total antral follicle count (AFC).

What do the hormonal tests of ovarian reserve mean?

Checking FSH levels can help assess a person's ovarian reserve. FSH is produced by the pituitary gland and plays a key role in stimulating the ovaries to mature eggs for ovulation. When ovarian reserve is low, the ovaries are less responsive, so the body compensates by producing higher levels of FSH. Therefore, an elevated FSH level, particularly measured on day 3 of the menstrual cycle, can indicate a reduced ovarian reserve. However, FSH is a hormone that continuously fluctuates throughout the menstrual cycle, so testing is usually repeated, and may be combined with other assessments to provide a more complete picture of fertility.

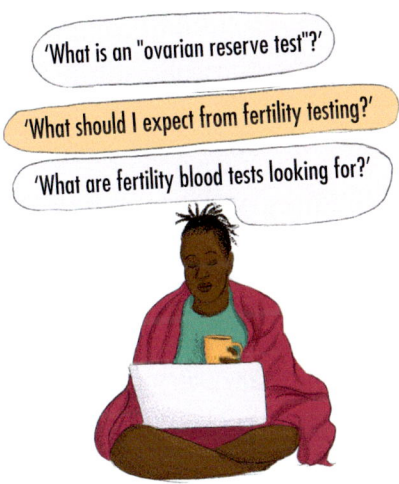

'What is an "ovarian reserve test"?'

'What should I expect from fertility testing?'

'What are fertility blood tests looking for?'

AMH is another hormone that can be tested. It is produced by the small developing follicles in the ovaries, so the amount of AMH in the blood reflects the number of these follicles. Higher AMH levels generally indicate a greater ovarian reserve (although very high levels can suggest PCOS), while lower levels suggest a reduced reserve.

Unlike other tests such as FSH, AMH levels remain relatively stable throughout the menstrual cycle, making it a more reliable marker that can be checked on any day of the cycle. Low AMH levels may indicate a decreased ovarian reserve, which can be associated with challenges in conceiving, but it does not directly reflect egg quality. Normal AMH levels are somewhere between 3 and 35.

DID YOU KNOW?

Am I fertile?

Recently, there has been a trend for women to have their 'fertility' checked using at-home test kits or specific blood tests marketed at well people who may be curious about whether they will have difficulty in conceiving. This is sometimes suggested to help people to determine if they are 'fertile', or if they should freeze their eggs or not. These kits, or private blood tests, often include checking ovarian reserve via AMH and FSH levels in healthy women without any specific fertility concerns.

It is important to remember that these tests were developed to inform IVF treatment and not to tell you if you will be able to fall pregnant in the future. Many women and people with ovaries who are told they have a low AMH level will conceive without any problems when they start actively trying, while others with a good ovarian reserve may take time and need fertility treatment.

There is no doubt that tests showing a good ovarian reserve are reassuring but they do not guarantee a baby. Equally, a poor or impaired ovarian reserve does not mean you will struggle and need fertility treatment.

When it comes to at-home fertility testing, it is a good idea to approach the idea with a healthy dose of scepticism. These factors may change over time, but currently at-home blood collection, which is often part of these tests, may not be as reliable as samples taken in a clinical setting, potentially leading to inaccurate results.

Additionally, many of the at-home tests focus on measuring AMH (anti-Müllerian hormone), which reflects ovarian reserve but does not determine whether someone is infertile, or how likely they are to conceive naturally. High or low AMH levels do not directly indicate fertility, and interpreting these results without professional guidance can lead to confusion or unnecessary worry.

Having blood tests to check your fertility might tell you something about your ovarian reserve, but it cannot be considered a full answer to the question 'Am I fertile?'. This is because it doesn't assess many other factors that affect fertility, like whether the fallopian tubes are blocked, the structure of the uterus, or the quality of your partner's sperm.

Therefore, I don't generally advise pursuing these ovarian reserve tests to check your fertility unless you and your doctor have already determined that fertility treatment is required. In this situation, ovarian reserve tests can be used to predict response to treatment and guide dosing of medications.

Age is, however, the ultimate marker of ovarian reserve, as we can be certain that the number and quality of eggs will decline over time.

Tubal tests

Tubal tests, such as a hysterosalpingography or saline sonography, are used to check if the fallopian tubes are open and functioning properly. These tests help identify blockages or structural issues that could prevent sperm from reaching the egg, impacting fertility.

Hysterosalpingography (HSG)

HSG is an X-ray procedure used to assess the uterus and fallopian tubes. During the test, a special dye is injected into the womb, and its movement is tracked on an X-ray screen to check if the dye flows freely through the fallopian tubes and out the ends, into the abdominal cavity. If the dye does not pass through, it may indicate a blockage or a temporary spasm in the tubes. HSG can also reveal any abnormalities in the shape of the uterine cavity and identify the site of any blockages in the tubes.

Hysterosalpingo-contrast sonography (HyCoSy)

HyCoSy is a procedure similar to HSG but uses ultrasound instead of X-rays to assess the uterus and fallopian tubes. A thin tube is inserted through the cervix, and a vaginal ultrasound provides real-time images on a screen as fluid is injected to show it filling the uterus and travelling through the fallopian tubes.

The main advantage of HyCoSy is that it can be done in an outpatient clinic without the need for X-ray equipment, avoiding radiation exposure – a common concern for those trying to conceive (though the small radiation dose from HSG is unlikely to cause harm even if someone is pregnant and doesn't realise it yet).

DID YOU KNOW?

Studies suggest that up to 30% of individuals conceive spontaneously within 6 months after HSG or HyCoSy.[7] This may be because the tubes get flushed with fluid, which can displace any mild non-obstructive blockages.

Laparoscopy

In some cases, if there are concerns about conditions affecting fertility, such as endometriosis or complications from a past pelvic infection, doctors may recommend keyhole surgery, also known as laparoscopy. This procedure is done under general anaesthesia, where a small incision is made near the belly button, and the abdomen is inflated with carbon dioxide to provide a clearer view of the pelvic organs. A thin camera, called a laparoscope, is inserted to inspect the uterus, ovaries, and fallopian tubes for issues like endometriosis or fibroids.

During the laparoscopy, a dye test can also be done to check if the fallopian tubes are open, similar to HSG or HyCoSy. If the tubes are clear, the dye will pass through them and exit from the outer openings.

Laparoscopy allows a direct view of the pelvic organs and thereby permits a much more accurate assessment, particularly to identify the presence of endometriosis. The majority of patients are able to leave the hospital the same day following a simple diagnostic laparoscopy. It is also possible to treat any issues identified at the same time, such as removing ovarian cysts, scar tissue, or mild–moderate endometriosis. If more severe endometriosis is identified, a follow-up surgery may be planned after more detailed discussion.

Hysteroscopy

Hysteroscopy is a procedure where a small camera is inserted through the cervix to examine the inside of the womb. The womb may be filled with carbon dioxide gas or fluid to help the doctor or nurse get a clear view. This procedure can be done with mild sedation and a local anaesthetic or under general anaesthesia, depending on the situation. It is an important tool for investigating structural issues in the womb that could cause problems, such as fibroids, polyps, extra walls dividing the uterine cavity, or adhesions (scar tissue) inside the uterus.

Male fertility tests

The basic fertility screening test for males, and people with a penis, is the semen analysis. In general, the lower the sperm count and the poorer the sperm quality, the longer it will take to conceive and the more difficult it may be for a pregnancy to occur.

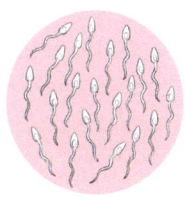

The male partner will be asked to produce a sample by means of masturbation directly into a special sterile container. It's important to keep the sample warm and deliver it to the laboratory within 1 hour of collection.

After the sample volume has been measured, the following calculations are carried out:

- **Sperm count:** The number of sperm per millilitre (ml)
- **Sperm motility:** The percentage of sperm that are moving and a description of their movement quality, ranging from good to non-motile

- **The percentage of abnormal sperm**
- **The number of white cells** in the sample is noted, as this may indicate infection

As sperm quality can vary significantly between samples, an abnormal semen analysis is usually followed by one or two repeat tests for confirmation.

The pathway of infertility treatment

The typical process for infertility treatment begins with initial tests to determine the underlying cause of infertility, as outlined earlier. After these tests, healthcare providers will discuss the results to pinpoint potential causes, such as ovulation disorders, fallopian tube blockages, or sperm issues. The course of treatment is then tailored to the specific cause of infertility and the individual's circumstances, ensuring a personalised approach.

Ovulation induction

If ovulation problems are identified, the first step may involve stimulating the ovaries to release the egg, in a process known as ovulation induction. Medications like clomiphene citrate or letrozole can be taken orally, usually for 5 days early in the menstrual cycle (typically starting on days 2–5). These medications stimulate the ovaries to mature and release eggs by increasing levels of certain reproductive hormones.

This treatment may be recommended if you have irregular periods, and the primary reason identified as a cause of subfertility is an issue with ovulation such as in conditions like PCOS. If you have regular periods, it is likely that ovulation is not the cause of your subfertility and so these medications are unlikely to be a helpful option.

Intrauterine insemination (IUI)

IUI is a fertility treatment where sperm are placed directly into the uterus to increase the chances of fertilisation. During the procedure, sperm are specially prepared and inserted into the uterus around the time of ovulation, which can either be spontaneous or induced by medications. The goal is to bring the sperm closer to the egg, bypassing any potential barriers in the cervix.

IUI may be suitable for individuals or couples with specific fertility challenges, such as mild male factor infertility, unexplained infertility, or cervical issues that prevent sperm from passing through. It's also a common choice for same-sex couples or single women using donor sperm.

However, IUI may not be suitable for individuals with certain conditions, such as severe male infertility, blocked fallopian tubes, or significant hormonal imbalances that affect ovulation. In these cases, more advanced treatments like IVF may be recommended.

In vitro fertilisation (IVF)

IVF is an assisted reproductive technology that involves fertilising an egg with sperm outside the body. This method is commonly used to overcome various fertility challenges, including fallopian tube blockages, low sperm count, endometriosis, or unexplained infertility.

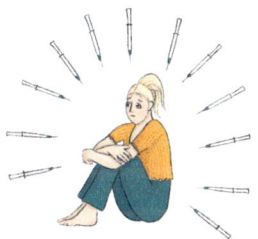

If you or someone you care about is planning to undergo IVF, here is what will happen as part of the process:

1. **Ovarian stimulation:** Fertility medications are given to stimulate the ovaries to mature multiple eggs at the same time. These are often given as a combination of injections, vaginal tablets, and oral medications on a daily basis for a period of around 2 weeks. During this time, the person will need to have multiple blood tests and scans to check how their body is responding

2. **Egg retrieval:** When the eggs are developing, an extra injection is then given to stimulate the final steps of maturation. Then, 24–48 hours later, a minor surgical procedure is performed. The procedure aims to retrieve mature eggs from the ovaries using a thin needle. This is called follicular aspiration. The doctor uses an ultrasound to guide a thin needle into each of the ovaries through the vagina. The needle has a device attached to it that suctions the eggs out one at a time. The egg

collection procedure is usually done while you are awake, but medications are available to reduce any discomfort and most people are able to go home the same day

3. **Sperm collection:** A sperm sample is collected, either from the male partner or a sperm donor. The sperm are then put through a high-speed wash and spin cycle in order to find the healthiest ones

4. **Fertilisation:** The eggs and sperm are combined in a laboratory dish, and fertilisation is monitored. It usually takes a few hours for a sperm to fertilise an egg and create an embryo. Intracytoplasmic sperm injection (ICSI) is sometimes performed as part of IVF to help with fertilisation. In ICSI, a single sperm is injected directly into an egg, instead of making the long journey along a fallopian tube. ICSI is particularly useful in cases of male factor infertility, such as low sperm count, poor sperm motility, or abnormal sperm shape. It's also used when previous IVF cycles have had poor fertilisation outcomes or when using frozen sperm or eggs. By injecting the sperm directly, ICSI increases the chances of fertilisation, especially in cases where sperm may struggle to fertilise the egg on their own

5. **Embryo culture:** Fertilised eggs (embryos) are cultured for a few days to allow development

Going through IVF can be an emotional rollercoaster, filled with moments of hope and excitement, but also significant emotional challenges. Throughout the IVF process, there is a natural drop-off in the number of eggs and embryos at each stage. For instance, if 15 eggs are retrieved, not all will mature – perhaps only 10. Not all of these will fertilise, leaving around six to eight embryos, and some may not continue developing, so by day 5, you might have only three or four high-quality embryos remaining for transfer or freezing. While it can be disheartening to see numbers decrease, it ultimately ensures that only the healthiest embryos are selected for transfer, providing the best possible chance for success

6. **Embryo transfer:** The next step requires progesterone to be given in order to prepare the lining of the uterus to receive the embryos. Over the 3–5 days, the embryos develop into blastocysts before they can be

transferred. The doctor will place the embryos in the uterus using a catheter. Like step number two, this part of IVF is usually performed while you are awake. Depending on the situation, one or multiple embryos are transferred back into the uterus in the hope that that at least one will implant itself and begin to develop. Sometimes more than one embryo ends up implanting, or the embryo may split after transfer, which is why multiple pregnancies are common in people who have IVF

7. **Luteal phase support:** Even after embryo transfer, the work isn't over. Hormonal medications are continued, which may involve injections or vaginal tablets, in order to support the uterine lining and early embryo development

8. **Pregnancy test:** 8–10 days after embryo transfer, a blood test can be arranged to determine whether the IVF cycle has resulted in pregnancy

At the end of an IVF cycle, emotions and physical experiences can vary greatly depending on the outcome and the individual's journey. If the result is positive, feelings of relief, excitement, and joy are common. However, if the cycle does not result in pregnancy, it can lead to disappointment, sadness, or frustration. Physically, many may feel drained from the hormonal treatments, egg retrieval, and embryo transfer. Additionally, the 2-week wait between transfer and pregnancy testing can heighten anxiety and emotional exhaustion. Regardless of the outcome, the process often leaves individuals reflecting on the emotional and physical toll IVF can take. Support from loved ones and a focus on self-care can help navigate this intense period.

Same-sex and single-parent relationships

Same-sex couples or individuals who wish to conceive have various fertility options available to them, depending on their preferences, circumstances, and medical considerations.

Here are some common fertility options for same-sex families:

1. **Intrauterine insemination (IUI):** IUI involves placing sperm directly into the uterus using a catheter. This can be a suitable option for female same-sex couples who choose to use donor sperm for conception:

- IUI is often used when there are no underlying fertility issues, and it is a less invasive and more affordable option compared to some other assisted reproductive technologies

2. **In vitro fertilisation (IVF):** IVF involves fertilising an egg with sperm outside the body and then implanting the embryo into the uterus:

   - For female same-sex couples or a single female parent, this would involve using donor sperm to create an embryo, and one of the partners with a uterus carrying the pregnancy to term

   - For a male same-sex couple or single parent, this would require donor eggs and a surrogate to carry the pregnancy

   - Surrogacy: This involves someone with a uterus carrying a pregnancy on behalf of another person or couple. Surrogacy can be a difficult option for same-sex couples due to a variety of legal, financial, and logistical challenges:

     o In many countries, surrogacy laws are complex and may not fully support same-sex couples, either prohibiting surrogacy entirely or making it hard for both partners to be recognised as legal parents

     o Additionally, the cost of surrogacy can be prohibitively high, as it often involves medical procedures, legal fees, and compensation for the surrogate. Finding a surrogate can also be challenging, and navigating the ethical and emotional complexities of the process adds further difficulties. These factors make surrogacy a complicated path for many same-sex couples

3. **Adoption:** Adoption is a non-biological option for building a family. It involves legally and permanently assuming parental rights for a child. Adoption provides a loving home to children in need and allows individuals or couples to become parents regardless of biological ties. However, it can also be a difficult option for same-sex couples due to legal restrictions in certain countries or regions, as well as societal biases that may favour heterosexual couples. Additionally, some adoption agencies may have policies that make the process more challenging for LGBTQ+ individuals, further complicating their path to adoption

1. EDUCATE YOURSELF ON THE PROCESS

Understanding the IVF process can help you feel more in control. While your clinic will guide you, waiting for your first appointment can feel long and sometimes frustrating. Use this time to research what IVF involves, including reading about common terms and what all the acronyms mean. Ask questions during appointments – there are no 'silly' questions when it comes to your health.

Knowledge empowers individuals to actively participate in decision-making and cope with the emotional aspects of the journey. It can also be helpful to speak to people you know who have been through the process, who may be able to signpost you to helpful resources and understand practically what you may need.

2. TAKE NOTES

Bring a notebook or ask to record appointments with your doctor. With so much information to absorb, it's easy to miss details or forget questions. Keeping a clear record can help you stay organised and ensure you understand every step.

3. CONSIDER TAKING TIME OFF

IVF can require time away from work, particularly around egg retrieval and embryo transfer. Consider discussing your needs with your employer in advance. Taking a few days off for physical recovery and emotional well-being can help you manage the demands of the process.

4. DISCUSS FLEXIBLE WORKING

Frequent scans and blood tests during the initial phase of IVF can be challenging to juggle with work. If possible, discuss flexible hours or remote working arrangements with your employer. This reduces stress and allows you to focus on your health without compromising your responsibilities. The easiest way to navigate this is to be open about what you are going through, and you will often find people are supportive. However, this might not be the case for everyone.

continued...

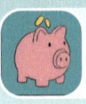 ## 5. BUDGETING FOR IVF

IVF costs vary significantly depending on treatment plans and location. Before starting, request a detailed breakdown of costs, including any additional procedures your doctor recommends. Explore options like payment plans, package deals, or fertility loans. It can take some time to save up or borrow the money needed to go through this process, which adds to the stress during an already difficult time.

The average number of IVF cycles needed to achieve a pregnancy varies, but research suggests that about 30–40% of IVF cycles result in a live birth. On average, it may take 2 to 3 cycles to achieve a pregnancy.[8] Success rates can depend on various factors such as age, underlying health conditions, and specific fertility issues. Since success often takes multiple cycles, prepare financially and emotionally for the possibility of needing more than one round.

 ## 6. MANAGING UNHELPFUL COMMENTS

Insensitive remarks from others can sting. When this happens, consider explaining how their words affected you, using 'I' statements to foster understanding, such as 'I know you meant well, but asking me when we are going to get on and have a baby was very upsetting'. Gentle education might not only stop future remarks but also help others support someone else in your position.

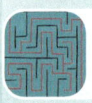 ## 7. BE FLEXIBLE

Fertility treatment is unpredictable, and your journey might not follow the original plan. By keeping your mind and your heart open to switching treatments or altering timelines, you are less likely to feel disappointed. Focus on the parts of the journey within your control and celebrate each little win along the way.

 ## 8. BUILD A SUPPORT SYSTEM

Not everyone wants to disclose that they are trying to conceive; they may be worried about implications at work, or they just don't want people asking them a million questions. However, IVF can feel isolating, and sharing your experience with trusted friends, family, or a support group can provide comfort. Some clinics also connect patients going through similar journeys. Even selective sharing can help you feel less alone.

 ## 9. PRIORITISE SELF-CARE

Protect your mental and physical health by engaging in activities that bring you joy and reduce stress. Whether it's exercising, meditating, or taking a break from family-focused gatherings, prioritise yourself during this finite period of time.

 ## 10. COMMUNICATE WITH YOUR PARTNER

IVF is an emotional experience for both partners. Openly sharing your feelings can strengthen your relationship and help you support each other through the highs and lows.

 ## 11. SEEK PROFESSIONAL SUPPORT

If you need it, don't hesitate to consult with a mental health professional or counsellor experienced in fertility issues. They can provide strategies for coping with stress and emotional challenges, especially if the process doesn't go the way you may have hoped.

 ## 12. STAY POSITIVE

Try to maintain a positive mindset. Celebrate small victories and milestones, and plan little treats for yourselves along the way, especially for the more difficult days. Maintain a focus on the end goal of parenthood but keep an open mind about how and when you may get there.

Remember, the journey through IVF is unique for each individual or couple.

How to support a loved one going through fertility treatment

Put yourself in their shoes

Consider texting instead of calling or announcing proudly at a celebratory dinner if you find out you are pregnant when you know your friend/sibling is struggling. It leaves the ball in their park and means you have given thought and awareness to their current situation. This will be really appreciated by the person going through it and respects their circumstances. Of course, you deserve joy and should be proud and excited with your happy news, but empathy really helps here.

If someone you care about is struggling, it is a good idea to avoid saying certain phrases like 'Oh, my friends were trying and then they just went on holiday and it happened' or 'Just relax and stop thinking about it.' You might be trying to be reassuring, but these words can have the opposite effect.

Ask if they're alright

If someone has announced a pregnancy in your friendship group, family, or at work, and you know another is struggling, you could message them to ask how they are doing, if they want to talk, or just offer to be there. It helps to know someone is thinking of you, while most of the attention is directed at the mum or dad to be. If they don't want to engage, don't push it – it's really nice to just offer.

Some helpful phrases are: 'I'm here for you if you need me' or 'I'm sorry you are going through this, it's rubbish, but I'm here.'

Offer to be there

If a loved one has shared their fertility journey with you, take the time to ask how involved they would like you to be. Some may want to discuss the process openly, while others might prefer limited conversation about it. Offer practical help, such as accompanying them to appointments or assisting with childcare if needed. Your willingness to acknowledge the physical and emotional demands of fertility treatment will make them feel seen and supported.

Support their choices

When someone is trying to conceive, they may adopt lifestyle changes – such as avoiding alcohol or cutting out certain foods – that might seem extreme or unnecessary to you. It's crucial to respect these decisions without judgement. They've likely done extensive research or are following professional advice. Avoid questioning their choices unless they ask for your opinion. Similarly, while it's natural to want to share advice or articles that you read, resist the urge to overwhelm them with unsolicited information. Trust that they are seeking the guidance they need.

Send them something nice!

Show your support with small, meaningful actions. If they're going through a tough time – like a failed treatment cycle, a miscarriage, or navigating triggers like other pregnancy announcements – a thoughtful gift, card, or flowers can brighten their day. Even simple gestures, such as offering to cook for them or bringing a takeout, can make a significant difference. The key is to remind them they're not alone and that you're thinking of them without expecting anything in return.

As shown in this chapter, fertility is not always as straightforward as we might be taught in school. There is plenty of help and support available but there is no denying that infertility is a cruel process, which can be emotionally, financially, and physically draining. As lonely and as isolating as it can feel, there are many others going through the journey alongside you, and finding someone you can speak to can make a huge difference. Take each day as it comes, and celebrate each little win along the way.

A history of contraception

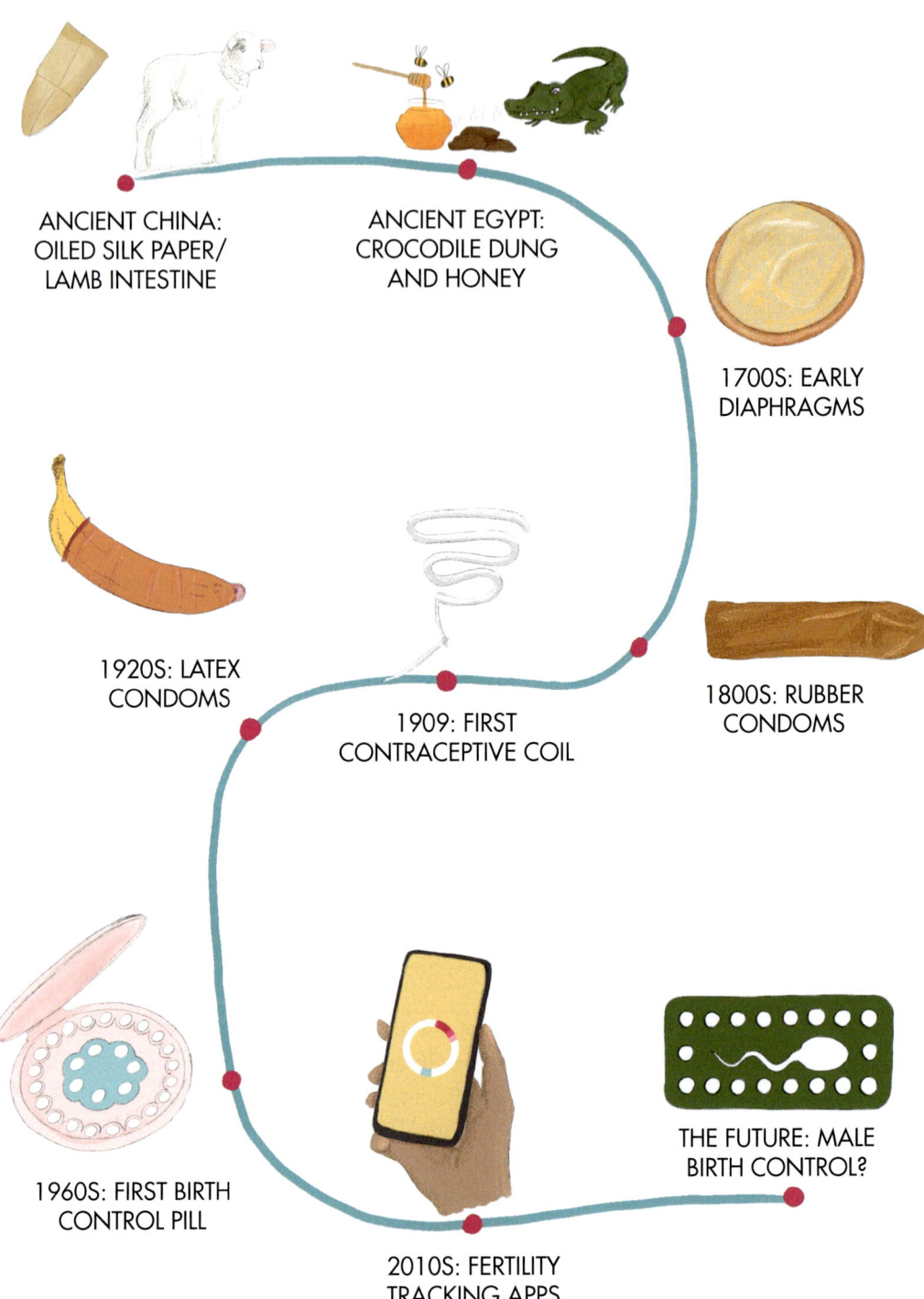

ANCIENT CHINA:
OILED SILK PAPER/
LAMB INTESTINE

ANCIENT EGYPT:
CROCODILE DUNG
AND HONEY

1700S: EARLY
DIAPHRAGMS

1920S: LATEX
CONDOMS

1909: FIRST
CONTRACEPTIVE COIL

1800S: RUBBER
CONDOMS

1960S: FIRST BIRTH
CONTROL PILL

2010S: FERTILITY
TRACKING APPS

THE FUTURE: MALE
BIRTH CONTROL?

CHAPTER 6

Contraception: not getting pregnant

Contraception as we know it is a modern innovation, but the desire to control fertility and enjoy sex without always resulting in a child is as old as humanity itself. Historical records show fascinating methods to prevent pregnancy: ancient Chinese civilisations used oiled silk or lamb intestine sheaths as barriers, while ancient Egyptians reportedly crafted pessaries from crocodile dung and honey. By the eighteenth century, early diaphragms were introduced, and the nineteenth century brought the popularisation of rubber condoms, which were more durable and effective than earlier materials.

The twentieth century, however, marked a revolution in family planning, with the development of hormonal contraception, including the approval of the birth control pill. These groundbreaking advancements have since expanded into a diverse array of options, from intrauterine devices (IUDs) to contraceptive patches, injections, and various formulations of oral contraceptives.

Today, modern contraception empowers individuals so they can choose to delay or space pregnancies or prevent conception entirely, offering safe, effective, and personalised choices. Beyond practicality, contraception has been transformative, liberating women to be able to control their reproductive journeys.

Hormonal versus non-hormonal contraception

Hormonal and non-hormonal contraception are the two main types of birth control, which work in different ways to prevent pregnancy.

Hormonal contraception

Hormonal methods of contraception involve the use of synthetic hormones, such as oestrogen and progestin. By changing hormone levels, these methods primarily work to prevent ovulation, change cervical mucus consistency, and modify the uterine lining to prevent fertilisation and implantation. These methods include oral contraceptives (birth control pills), hormonal patches, injections, and hormonal intrauterine devices (IUDs).

Hormonal birth control methods are popular but they can cause side effects like mood changes, bloating, and irregular bleeding, which some people find difficult to tolerate. Others may not be suitable for hormonal options due to health risks, so hormone-free alternatives can be a better fit for their needs and preferences.

Non-hormonal contraception

Non-hormonal methods of contraception use various mechanisms to create blockages to the passage of sperm, prevent sperm mobility, or disrupt fertilisation. Examples include barrier methods like condoms, diaphragms, and cervical caps, as well as fertility awareness methods and copper-based intrauterine devices (IUDs). There are also more permanent methods of preventing pregnancy, such as sterilisation procedures or removal of the uterus (hysterectomy).

There are some questions you can ask yourself to help you choose which method is right for you.

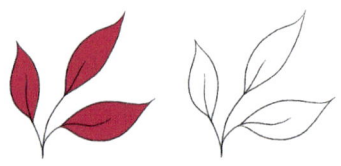

Which contraception is right for you?

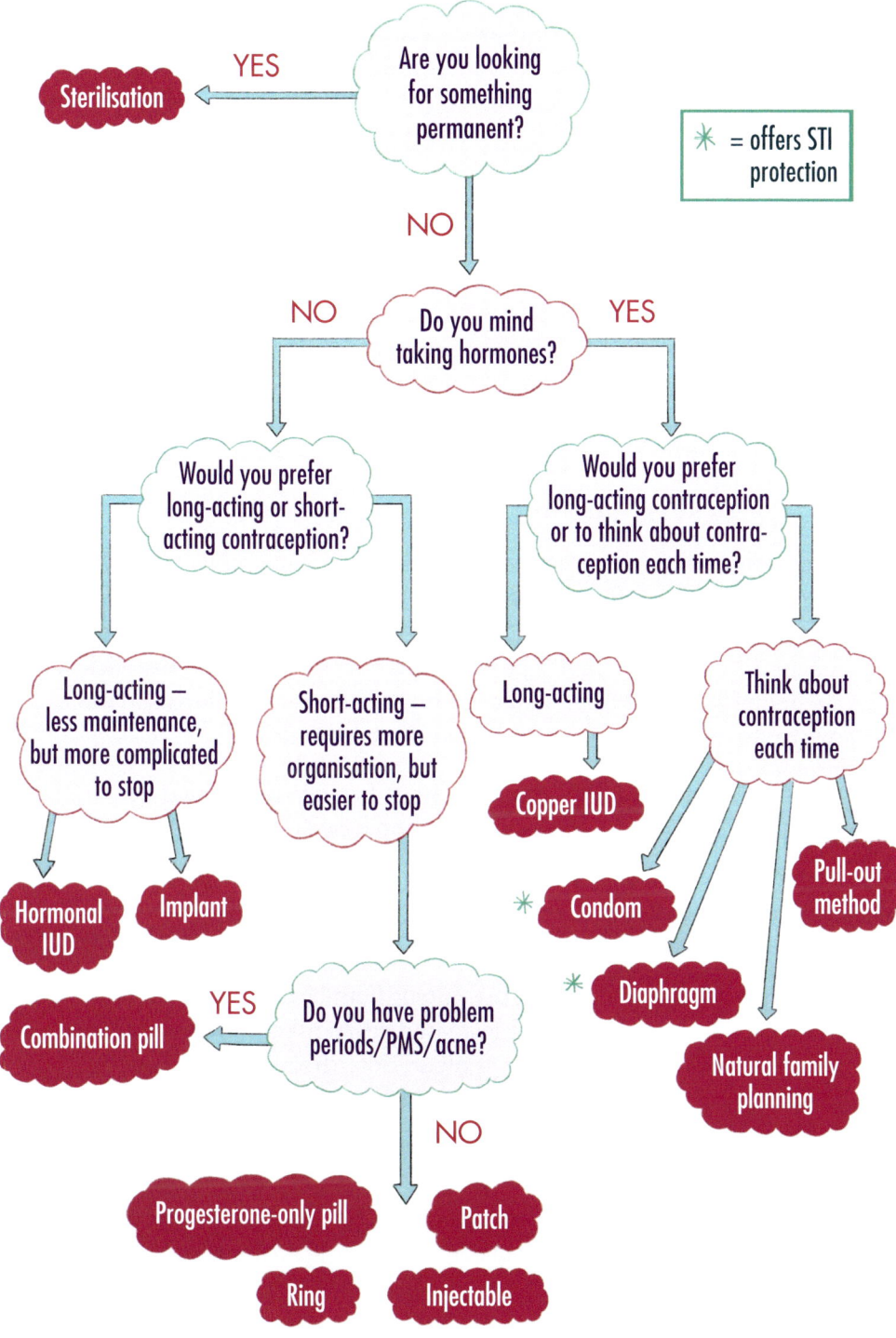

Are your periods an issue?

Hormonal contraceptives often have the additional benefit of improving painful, heavy, or irregular periods while preventing pregnancy at the same time. Consider bringing a menstrual diary to your appointment when you are discussing contraception so you can work out which is the best choice for you.

Are you planning a pregnancy soon?

If your family is complete or you don't plan to have children, you might opt for semi-permanent or permanent contraception. A copper IUD provides hormone-free, long-term protection for up to 10 years and can be removed anytime, while sterilisation offers a permanent solution. On the other hand, if you may be thinking about conceiving in the next few months you may opt for a method that is short-lasting and simple to reverse, such as condoms or the contraceptive pill.

Does the idea of taking hormones bother you?

If you are seeking a more 'natural' route, then you might prefer to opt for one of the hormone-free options. It is important not to demonise the idea of taking hormones, because they can be a fantastic option where needed for controlling and improving period symptoms. However, alternatives that are free from synthetic hormones also do have fewer side effects and can be quicker to reverse, which may suit some lifestyles better.

How old are you, and how far are you away from the menopause?

Depending on your age, your doctor may guide you away from certain types of hormonal contraception such as the combined pill, but this doesn't mean you can't have any hormonal contraception at all.[1]

Doctors may be cautious about prescribing hormonal contraception to those over the age of 35, due to increased health risks. As women age, the risk of cardiovascular issues, such as blood clots, stroke, and heart attack, rises. Hormonal contraceptives, particularly those containing oestrogen, can further increase these risks, although they can be reduced by giving the hormones via a different route, such as via the skin instead of as oral tablets.

If you are closer to the menopause, and your family is complete, you may also prefer longer-acting forms of contraception, like a hormonal coil, which will also benefit you if you experience some of the changes in bleeding pattern that can occur when you approach the menopause.

Are you likely to achieve 'perfect' use?

Methods like fertility awareness, where people track their cycle, temperature, and other factors to help determine when they are most fertile are great for helping you understand your body. However, not everyone can be absolutely consistent daily with these tasks. If you don't always wake up at the same time or prefer to be more spontaneous when it comes to sex with a partner, then you may prefer methods that are less dependent on you remembering about certain tasks each day!

DID YOU KNOW?

Currently, hormonal contraception is only licensed for use by women, and people with a uterus, to prevent pregnancy.

There has been research into hormonal contraception for males, primarily focusing on suppressing sperm production through hormone regulation. However, it has been challenging due to the need to suppress millions of sperm produced daily, compared to the single egg targeted in female contraception. Making male contraception consistently effective, with few side effects, and available in easy-to-use forms like a daily pill has been difficult to achieve. Additionally, trust issues arise – many women may feel hesitant to rely on men to remember to take contraception daily when women bear the consequences of unintended pregnancies. Economic and regulatory hurdles further slow progress, as pharmaceutical companies are cautious about investing in methods that might not meet high demand or approval standards.

Therefore, at the time of writing, no male birth control method has yet been licenced for use.

Hormonal contraception – which is right for me?

Choosing the right hormonal contraception depends on your individual needs and goals, which we'll explore in detail later. Most hormonal options (whether progesterone-only or combined) work by:

1. Thickening cervical mucus to block sperm from reaching the egg
2. Stopping ovulation, so no egg is released for fertilisation
3. Thinning the uterine lining, making it less suitable for implantation

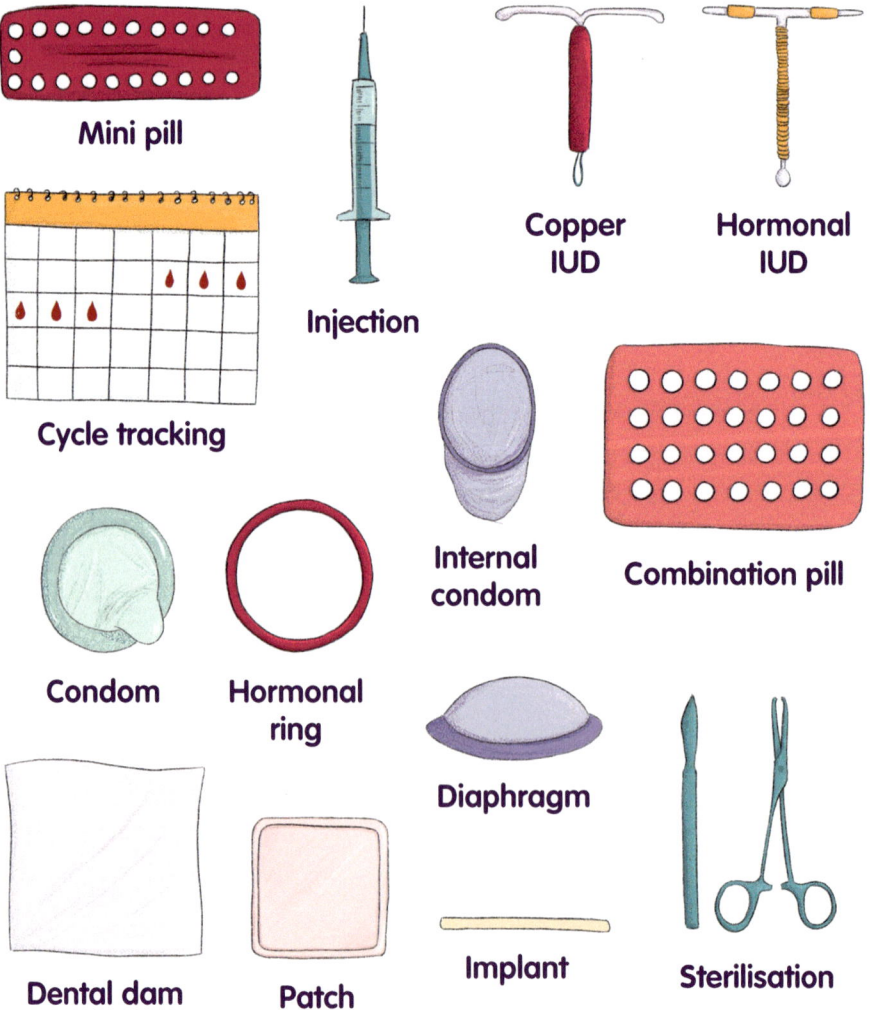

Mini pill

Cycle tracking

Injection

Copper IUD

Hormonal IUD

Condom

Hormonal ring

Internal condom

Combination pill

Dental dam

Patch

Diaphragm

Implant

Sterilisation

DID YOU KNOW?

When you have a bleed while taking hormonal contraception, this isn't called a period!

A withdrawal bleed occurs when you take a break from the active hormones (typically during the pill-free or the placebo week). This break causes a drop in hormone levels, mimicking the natural decline of hormones that triggers a period. However, this bleed is not a true period because ovulation hasn't occurred, and the bleeding is usually lighter.

Progesterone-only options

Progesterone-only contraceptive options refer to birth control methods that contain only the hormone progesterone (or its synthetic form, progestin, also known as progestogen), without any oestrogen.

Common progesterone-only contraceptive options include:

1. **Progesterone-only pills (POPs),** also known as the mini-pill, taken daily

2. **Hormonal IUDs** (e.g., Mirena), which release small amounts of synthetic progesterone into the uterus continuously

3. **Contraceptive implants** (e.g., Nexplanon), which are inserted under the skin and provide long-term contraception

4. **Contraceptive injections** (e.g., Depo-Provera), which are administered every 3 months

The progesterone-only pill (POP)

This contains a synthetic form of progesterone, which thickens your cervical mucus to prevent sperm from reaching an egg, therefore preventing pregnancy. Certain types of POP can also work by stopping ovulation.

The POP needs to be taken once a day, every day, to work and there are usually 28 pills supplied in each blister pack. There is no break between packs, so as soon as one finishes, you go straight on to start the next pack the next day.

There are two main types of POP – the 3-hour window POP (the traditional POP) and the 12-hour window POP (the desogestrel POP, e.g., Cerazette). Knowing which type of pill you are taking is important because the POP is only reliable as contraception if taken at approximately same time every day, which can be difficult depending on your lifestyle.

Top tip: When you start your first pack, choose a time of the day convenient to you and set a discreet alarm on your phone to get yourself into the habit.

The benefits of the POP are that, when taken correctly, it is more than 99% effective at preventing pregnancy.[2] Unlike combined hormonal contraceptives, the POP contains no oestrogen, making it a safer alternative for individuals with health conditions such as a history of blood clots, migraines with aura, or breast cancer. It is also an excellent choice for breastfeeding individuals, as it does not affect milk supply.

DID YOU KNOW?

The quoted effectiveness of contraception (such as 99% effective for the pill) is often based on 'perfect use' in scientific studies. This means the medication is taken exactly as prescribed, with no missed doses and under ideal conditions. However, in the 'real world', people might forget to take a pill, miss doses, or use contraception inconsistently, which leads to a lower effectiveness rate. This is known as the 'typical use' effectiveness.

For example, oral contraceptive pills may have a perfect use efficacy of over 99%, but in real-world settings, the effectiveness drops to around 91% due to user error. In studies, participants are often closely monitored and follow strict guidelines, while in everyday life, human error and lifestyle factors come into play, impacting the actual success rate of the contraception.

POP – over 99% effective when taken effectively

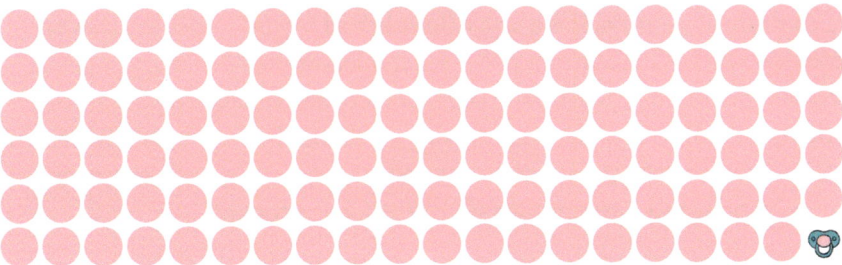

POP – 91% effective with typical use

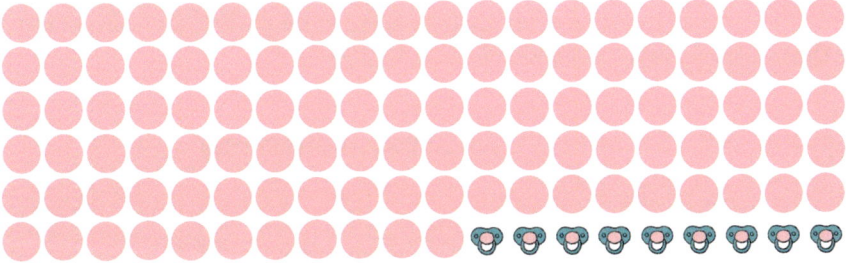

In addition to its safety profile, the POP can positively influence menstrual patterns. Many users experience lighter or less frequent periods, and for some, bleeding may stop altogether, providing relief for those with heavy or painful menstruation. While some initial irregular bleeding or spotting is common as the body adjusts, most people find their bleeding stabilises within a few months.

The main drawback of the POP is the need for strict daily timing; missing or delaying a dose increases the risk of pregnancy. Irregular or unscheduled bleeding, known as spotting, is another common issue and can be unpredictable, disrupting daily life. While this often improves with continued use, it may persist for some individuals. Other side effects include acne, mood changes, and breast tenderness, which are usually more noticeable in the first few months and tend to settle over time.

The progesterone implant (e.g., Nexplanon)

The contraceptive implant is a small, flexible rod placed under the skin of the upper arm by a healthcare provider. It releases the hormone progestin into the bloodstream, preventing pregnancy by thickening cervical mucus, stopping ovulation, and thinning the uterine lining. This low-maintenance method provides effective contraception for up to 3 years, offering a long-term solution without requiring daily or frequent attention.

One of the implant's major benefits is its reliability and convenience. Once inserted, it provides continuous contraception but also can be easily reversed, allowing fertility to return quickly after removal, often within 1–3 months. Many users also experience lighter periods or even find their bleeding stops all together after a while. This can be a significant advantage for those seeking relief from heavy or painful periods.

Implant – 99.95% effective when taken effectively

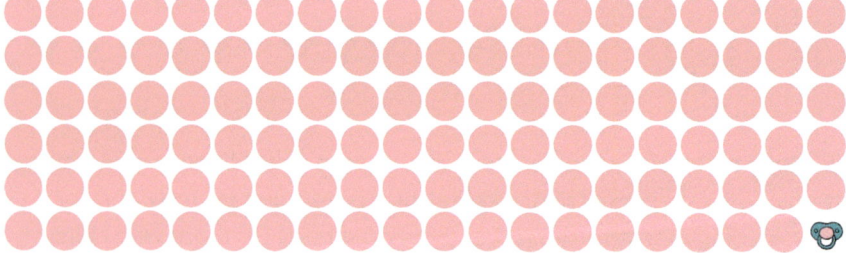

Implant – 99.95% effective when taken typically

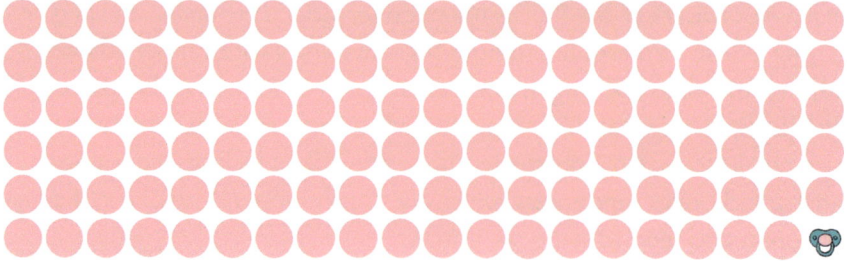

The main disadvantages are that the implant requires a minor surgical procedure for both insertion and removal. While these procedures are relatively simple, they can be uncomfortable and require a healthcare provider.

The commonest reason people ask for the implant to be removed is because they experience irregular or unpredictable vaginal bleeding. The data suggest that this is likely to improve over time, and after 6 months, 20% of users eventually have no bleeding at all but 50% continue to have some unpredictable bleeding.[3] Other side effects which are common to all progesterone-containing contraceptives are headaches, breast tenderness, or mood changes. These effects vary among individuals, and not everyone will experience them.

The depot progesterone injection (e.g., Depo-Provera)

The contraceptive injection works by releasing a synthetic form of the hormone progestin (medroxyprogesterone acetate) into the body. The injection prevents pregnancy for around 12 weeks (3 months), and after this period, hormone levels in the body drop and the injection's effectiveness decreases. To maintain continuous contraception and prevent ovulation, a repeat injection is required every 3 months. Missing or delaying the injection increases the risk of pregnancy. With perfect use, it is 99% effective, though with typical use – where some miss their scheduled doses – it is around 94% effective.

The injection offers several benefits, including reduced menstrual symptoms like lighter or absent periods, making it particularly useful for those with troublesome periods. It is discreet, requiring no daily pills or visible markers of use. It's also convenient for those who prefer a method they don't have to think about daily or weekly.

However, there are drawbacks to consider. Firstly, using the contraceptive injection can lead to a prolonged return to your baseline level of fertility. This is because after discontinuing the depot injection, it may take up to 9 months for your periods to restart and become regular, and it may even take up to 2 years for your fertility to return to normal. Some users experience side effects like weight gain, mood changes, or irregular bleeding. Regular 3-monthly appointments for injections can also be a challenge for some users. Long-term use may decrease bone density, especially in those with risk factors like smoking or steroid use, so it is recommended that after 2 years you review your contraceptive choices with your doctor to see if there is another more suitable alternative or whether it is safe to continue.

Injection – 99% effective when used correctly

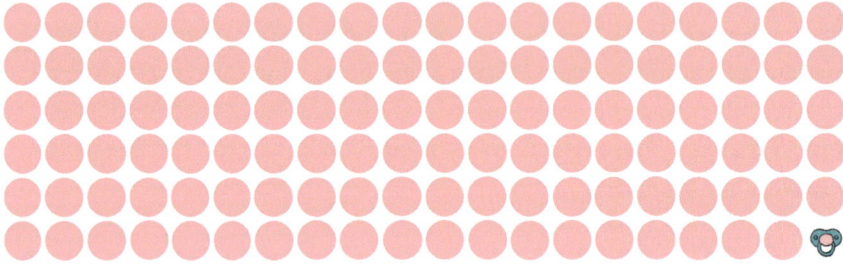

Injection – 94% effective with typical use

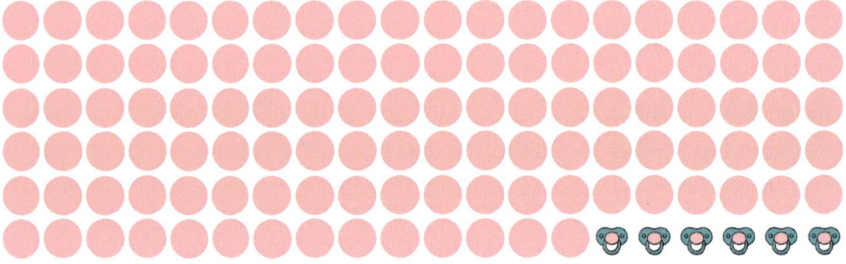

Combined hormonal contraception

When combined hormonal contraception (CHC) was first developed in the 1950s, it was originally intended to alleviate menstrual cycle symptoms. By the 1960s, however, it was marketed as a birth control method, sparking societal and moral debates about its role in family planning. The introduction of hormonal contraception marked a turning point in the fabric of society, allowing women to take control over their reproductive choices. This new availability ignited political discussions, particularly around whether it should be provided to both married and unmarried women.

Over time, access to the pill has dramatically transformed society, offering women the ability to decide when or if they want to have children. This autonomy has enabled many to pursue careers, become more financially in-dependent, and play a more prominent role in the workforce. Furthermore, it has contributed to significant shifts in sexual freedom, enabling people to engage in sexual activity for reasons beyond procreation.

CHC contains both progesterone and oestrogen and includes methods like the combined pill, the contraceptive patch, and the vaginal ring. These work together to prevent pregnancy in three main ways:

1. **Inhibiting ovulation:** Oestrogen and progesterone stop the ovaries from releasing eggs each month

2. **Thickening cervical mucus:** Progesterone makes the mucus in the cervix thicker, which blocks sperm from entering the uterus

3. **Thinning the uterine lining:** This makes it less likely for a fertilised egg to implant and grow

COCP – over 99.7% effective when taken effectively

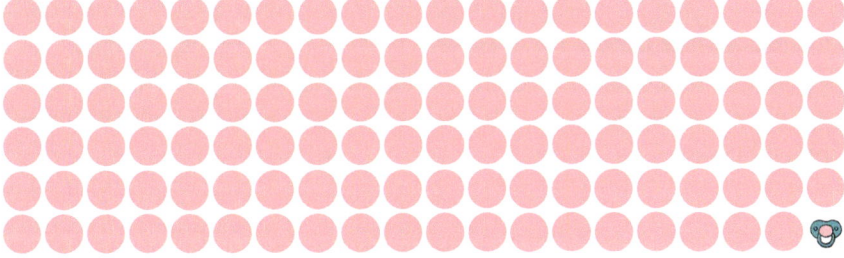

COCP – 91% effective with typical use

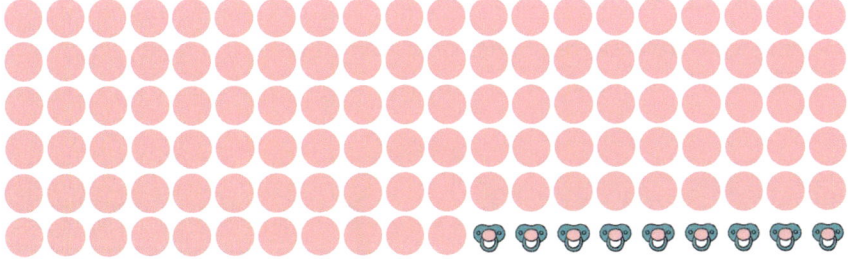

The oestrogen component offers additional benefits by stabilising the uterine lining, to reduce irregular or breakthrough bleeding and enhancing the overall effectiveness of contraception by more thoroughly preventing ovulation.

There are many different subtypes of CHC, with each containing different combination or amounts of hormones, and they may also be given different names in different countries.

- **Combined pill:** Taken daily, this oral medication (traditionally known as 'the pill') is available in 21-day or 28-day packs (with some pills being inactive). The variety of hormone doses and types on the market mean that doctors can offer patients different versions if one type doesn't suit

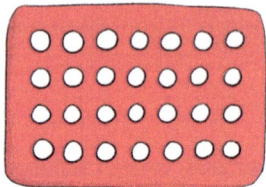

- **Contraceptive patch:** These are skin patches applied and changed every few days, which release hormones through the skin. They are usually worn for 3 weeks, with a patch-free week during which time a withdrawal bleed occurs

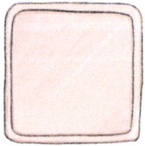

- **Vaginal ring:** This is a small, flexible ring inserted into the vagina for 3 weeks, which releases hormones close to the uterus. It is removed for a week every month to allow for a breakthrough bleed before the next cycle

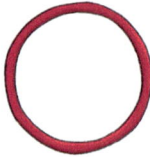

The combined pill

There are several different methods of taking the combined pill. The combined oral contraceptive pill (COCP) was originally designed to be taken in a way that was more 'acceptable' to society, by making it simulate the 'natural' menstrual cycle by giving a bleed every 4 weeks. That way, it was thought to improve compliance, but it also meant women didn't necessarily have to tell their husbands that they were taking it because they would still be having a bleed at the usual time!

This method is still frequently used today, and has the benefit of giving a predictable, regular monthly bleed. However, it is also worth knowing that the withdrawal bleed isn't strictly necessary. See below!

Traditional method

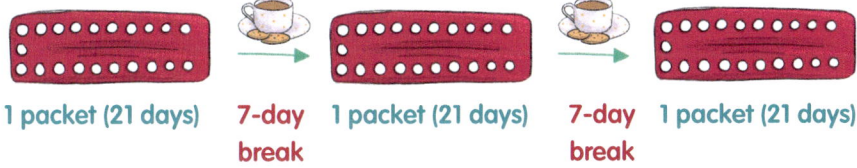

1 packet (21 days) 7-day break 1 packet (21 days) 7-day break 1 packet (21 days)

Traditional method

The traditional method of taking the COCP involves taking the pill daily for 21 consecutive days followed by a 7-day break when no pills are taken and a withdrawal bleed occurs. This bleed may start a few days after the 7-day break begins, and is likely to be shorter and lighter than your usual period.

After the 7-day break, a new pack of pills is started on the 8th day, even if the withdrawal bleed hasn't stopped. This cycle of 21 days of active pills followed by a 7-day break is repeated each month. Some formulations include 28-day packs where 7 pills are placebos (inactive) to help maintain the habit of daily pill taking without an actual hormone-free break.

Tricycling

The tricycling method of taking the COCP involves extending the pill-taking phase by taking three packs of active pills back-to-back without a break. After taking the pills continuously for 63 days (3 months), a 7-day break is taken, during which a withdrawal bleed occurs. This reduces the frequency

Tricycling

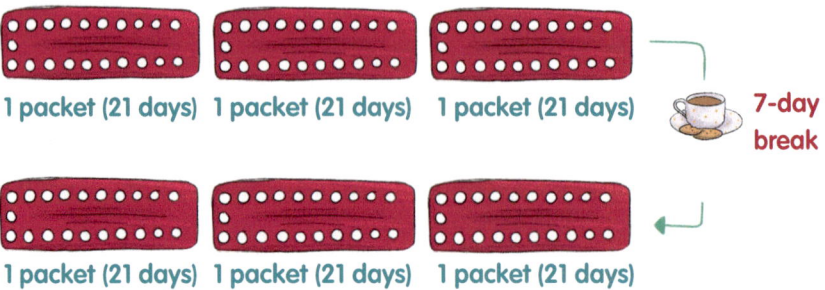

1 packet (21 days)   1 packet (21 days)   1 packet (21 days)   **7-day break**

1 packet (21 days)   1 packet (21 days)   1 packet (21 days)

of withdrawal bleeds to once every 3 months instead of every month, which some people find more convenient, especially if you are travelling or your bleeds are usually quite heavy or painful!

The break doesn't always need to be taken every 3 months, as the pill can sometimes be taken for longer periods (or shorter, depending on individual needs and medical advice).

Continuous pill taking*

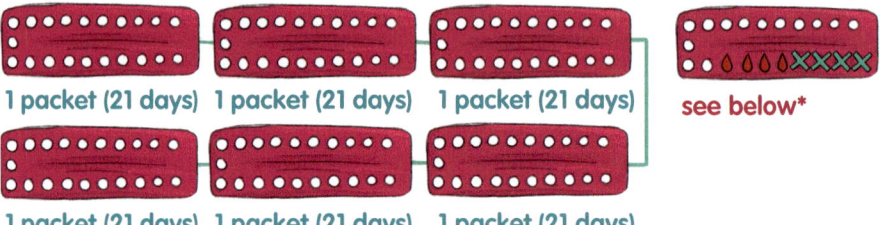

1 packet (21 days)   1 packet (21 days)   1 packet (21 days)   **see below***

1 packet (21 days)   1 packet (21 days)   1 packet (21 days)

*If you bleed for 4 days in a row, then it is recommended that you stop taking your pills for 4–7 days before restarting to allow the bleeding to continue, and then start taking the pills again. This is a more tailored way of giving yourself a pill-free interval when your body needs it and reduces the chances of you having breakthrough bleeding at other times. You should not take a break more than once every 4 weeks, or this could affect your contraception.

Continuous pill taking

The continuous method of taking the COCP involves taking the active hormone pills every day without any breaks or placebo pills. This means that you don't have a scheduled withdrawal bleed and, as a result, menstrual bleeding is either greatly reduced or eliminated altogether. The continuous method can be beneficial for those who want to avoid the inconvenience of regular periods or for managing conditions like endometriosis or severe menstrual cramps.

While many people may not experience any bleeding when using the continuous method, breakthrough bleeding (unexpected bleeding or spotting) can sometimes occur. This is generally normal and tends to decrease over time as the body adjusts to continuous hormone use.

DID YOU KNOW?

You are still protected from pregnancy during a pill-free break using the continuous method, as long as you've taken the pills correctly leading up to the break and it doesn't exceed 7 days.

However, if you decide to take a break longer than 7 days, protection from pregnancy could be compromised so you should use additional contraception if you do not wish to conceive. After any pill-free break, it is important to resume taking the pill on time to maintain contraceptive effectiveness.

Pros and cons of combined hormonal contraception

Benefits of CHC:

- **Highly effective:** CHC is 99% effective when used correctly, offering reliable contraception without disrupting intimacy

- **Convenient:** Once the pill is in your system, you don't need to think about contraception before sexual activity

- **More flexible use:** Although consistency is key, CHC offers more flexibility than the progesterone-only pill (POP) regarding the timing of doses. A few hours' variation won't significantly impact its effectiveness

- **Additional benefits:** The oestrogen component in CHC can improve acne for some women, relieve premenstrual syndrome (PMS), and may reduce the risk of ovarian, uterine, and colon cancers[4]

Disadvantages of CHC:

- **Side effects:** Some users may experience headaches, nausea, mood changes, and breast tenderness

- **Breakthrough bleeding:** Spotting can occur, especially in the first few months of use, though this usually improves over time

- **Slightly increased breast cancer risk:** Some studies suggest a minor increase in the risk of breast cancer while using CHC. However, this risk decreases once the contraceptive is stopped, and by 10 years after discontinuation, the risk returns to the same level as those who have never used CHC[5]

- **Increased risk of blood clots:** CHC slightly raises the risk of developing blood clots, especially in smokers, those over 35, or individuals with a history of blood clots. Therefore, CHC may not be suitable for people with specific health issues like migraines, blood clotting disorders, or a history of certain cancers or liver disease. The pill can be given at any age, but for individuals over 40, doctors suggest discussing other contraceptive options to see if there is a more suitable alternative[6]

What if you forget a pill?

While it's not critical to take the COCP at the exact same time every day, it is recommended to take it around the same time for maximum effectiveness and to reduce the risk of forgetting a pill. This helps maintain consistent hormone levels in your body, which is crucial for preventing ovulation and providing reliable contraception.

If you're late in taking the pill by a few hours, your protection typically remains intact, especially with COCP, which contains both oestrogen and progesterone and remains effective if taken within a 24-hour window. If you miss a pill for 24 hours or more, the effectiveness might be reduced so you should follow the missed pill rules for your pill type.

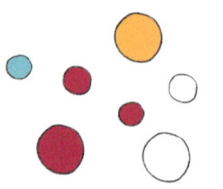

In summary...

Both the POP and COCP are short-acting methods of the contraceptive pill that are extremely effective when used correctly. The hormone content differs between the two, so if for whatever reason you aren't suitable to have the COCP, the POP is usually a safe alternative.

However, it is a commitment to remember to take your pill at roughly the same time every day. If you miss your pills and do not remember to take your next one within a suitable window, you risk having an unplanned pregnancy. If you can't commit to this, you may prefer to consider a long-acting method of contraception such as the coils, implants, or injection.

Some people also dislike the idea that they do not have periods while they take the hormonal contraception; as you do not ovulate, if you experience any bleeding this is called a withdrawal bleed. Although these bleeds are healthy, if you prefer to observe your natural menstrual cycle, then it may be better to choose a hormone-free method of contraception.

Non-hormonal contraception

Condoms

A short history of condoms

Condoms, as a form of barrier contraception, have a long history. The earliest known evidence of condom use dates back to ancient civilisations, with materials like linen sheaths or animal bladders employed for protection. However, the more recognisable rubber condom emerged in the mid-nineteenth century. Technological advancements have led to the development of latex condoms, which are widely used today for their effectiveness in preventing both unintended pregnancies and sexually transmitted infections (STIs).

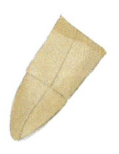 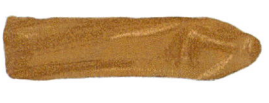 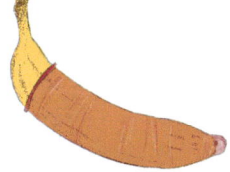

CONDOM GUIDE

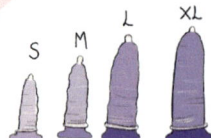

CORRECT FIT: Choosing the right size is crucial for effectiveness and comfort. Condoms come in various sizes, so individuals should experiment to find the one that fits securely without being too tight or too loose.

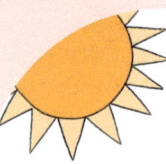
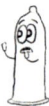

STORAGE: Condoms should be stored in a cool, dry place away from sunlight. Exposure to heat, moisture, and light can weaken the latex and reduce the effectiveness of the condom.

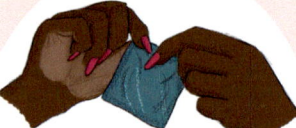

CHECK EXPIRY DATE: Always check the expiration date before using a condom. Expired condoms may be less effective and more prone to breakage.

OPEN CAREFULLY: When opening the condom wrapper, use care to avoid tearing the condom. Be mindful of sharp objects like fingernails or jewellery.

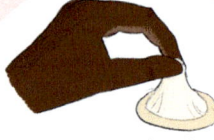

PINCH THE TIP: Before rolling the condom onto the erect penis, pinch the tip to leave a small reservoir. This space is essential to collect semen, preventing the condom from bursting through ejaculation.

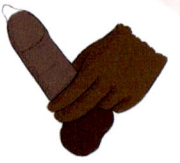

ROLL CAREFULLY: Roll the condom down the shaft of the penis until it is fully unrolled. Ensure it covers the entire length, leaving no exposed areas.

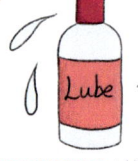

USE LUBRICATION: Adding water-based or silicone lubricant can enhance comfort and reduce the risk of breakage. However, avoid oil-based lubricants, as they can weaken the latex.

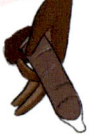

REMOVE CAREFULLY: After ejaculation and before losing an erection, withdraw the penis carefully while holding the base of the condom to prevent slippage.

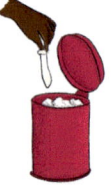

DISPOSE PROPERLY: After use, tie a knot at the open end of the condom to avoid spillage, and dispose of it in a trash bin.

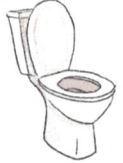

Avoid flushing condoms down toilets, as they can contribute to plumbing issues.

Condoms play a vital role in promoting safe and responsible sexual practices. When used consistently and correctly, they provide effective protection against both pregnancy and STIs, making them an essential tool for individuals and couples seeking reliable contraception.

Natural family planning methods

Natural family planning involves methods that help individuals or couples determine fertile and non-fertile periods within a woman's menstrual cycle, allowing them to make informed decisions about when to engage in sexual activity based on their family planning goals.

The following are different methods of natural family planning.

Fertility awareness-based methods

These methods rely on tracking signs of fertility to avoid intercourse or use barrier methods during fertile days.

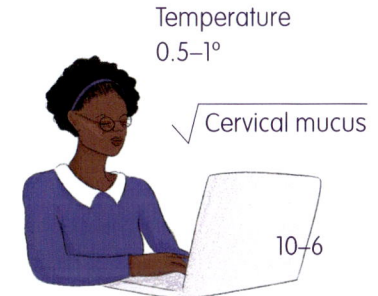

Temperature
0.5–1°

Cervical mucus

10–6

1. **Calendar method:** This involves tracking menstrual cycle dates to estimate the fertile window (typically days 10–16 of a regular cycle). It's less reliable for people with irregular cycles, as predicting fertile days based on dates alone can be inaccurate

2. **Basal body temperature (BBT):**
    By taking your temperature every morning before getting out of bed, you can detect a slight rise (0.5–1°C) that occurs after ovulation. Since sperm can survive in the body for a few days, avoid intercourse from several days before the temperature rise until about 4 days after. This method requires consistency and is best suited to those who can maintain a regular routine

3. **Cervical mucus method:** Fertile mucus, which is clear, stretchy, and slippery (similar to egg whites), signals ovulation. The mucus appears different throughout the month, and monitoring the changes can help identify fertile days. However, many factors can affect how the mucus looks, so it may not be a foolproof indicator of your fertile window. (More about these changes in Chapter 4 on hormones!)

4. **Symptothermal method:** This combines the calendar, BBT, and cervical mucus methods for greater accuracy. Apps and technology now support tracking these indicators, and can provide notifications or reminders. Over 1 year, fewer than 1 in 100 women would be expected to fall pregnant with perfect use of the symptothermal method, although this drops to 86% with imperfect use[7]

While these methods are hormone-free and natural, they require careful monitoring, consistency, and good knowledge of your cycle to be effective. Therefore, they are helpful for knowing that you should have sex now, when you are trying to conceive. If you want to avoid pregnancy, make sure you avoid sex during the suggested fertile window.

Lactational amenorrhea method

This method relies on breastfeeding as a natural contraceptive. It is most effective when a woman exclusively breastfeeds, and her menstrual cycle has not resumed.

For the method to be most reliable, all the following must apply:

- No period since birth
- Baby younger than 6 months
- Baby feeding from the breast frequently day and night, with gaps no longer than 4 hours
- Baby is exclusively breastfed (no feeds substituted for formula or expressed milk)
- Not yet weaned onto solids
- No dummies or bottles as this can reduce the time spent suckling at the breast

If any of these factors do not apply, there may be times in the day that your prolactin levels drop, meaning you may begin ovulating at any point. Therefore, if you do not wish to conceive, you may prefer to choose another alternative form of contraception which is safe when breastfeeding (discussed later in this chapter).

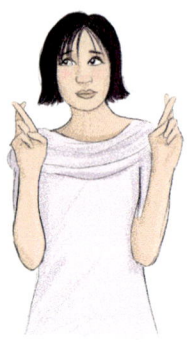

Pull-out method (withdrawal)

The pull-out method involves the withdrawing of the penis from the vagina before ejaculation to prevent sperm from entering the reproductive tract. While it's hormone-free and requires no devices, it has a typical effectiveness of around 78%, meaning 22 out of 100 people using it as their primary method of contraception may become pregnant in a year.[8] The presence of pre-ejaculate (pre-cum) can reduce the effectiveness of the withdrawal method of contraception. Pre-ejaculate may contain sperm from previous ejaculations, which can lead to pregnancy even if full ejaculation occurs outside the vagina.

While it is a form of natural family planning, it is considered less reliable than other methods and has a higher risk of unintended pregnancy.

Pull-out method – 78% effective with typical use

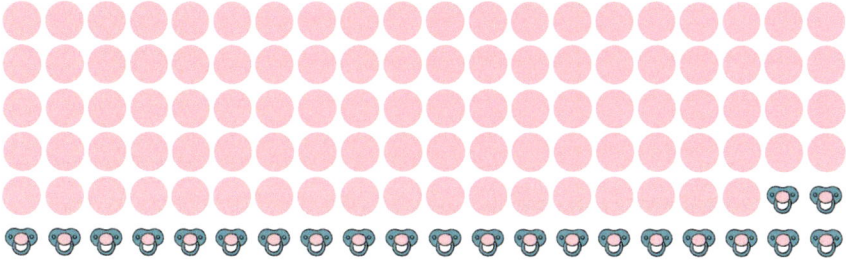

Are natural family planning methods right for you?

Natural family planning requires commitment, consistency, and a clear understanding of your fertility signs. It works best for those with regular cycles who are highly motivated to track their fertility accurately. While it can be empowering and hormone-free, it's less reliable than other methods. If you're okay with the small risk of pregnancy, it might suit you. However, if avoiding pregnancy is crucial, a more reliable and low-maintenance option may be a better fit.

Sterilisation

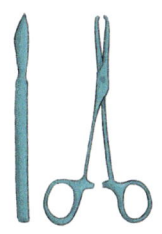

Sterilisation is a permanent, hormone-free contraceptive option that involves surgical procedures to permanently prevent pregnancy. It is suitable for individuals who are certain they do not wish to have biological children in the future or who have other health or personal reasons for choosing a permanent method.

For women and people with ovaries, sterilisation is typically performed through a procedure called tubal ligation. This involves blocking or sealing the fallopian tubes, either by tying and cutting them or by using clips or rings, preventing eggs from traveling from the ovaries to the uterus.

For men and people with testes, sterilisation is achieved through vasectomy, which involves cutting and sealing the vas deferens, the tubes that carry sperm from the testicles to the urethra. This prevents sperm from mixing with semen during ejaculation.

Sterilisation is excellent at preventing pregnancy; at over 99% effective, it is similar to other forms of contraception like coils and pills. Male sterilisation (vasectomy) is actually a more reliable procedure, with fewer than 1 in 1,000 unintended pregnancies after the procedure, compared with a failure rate of less than 1 in 100 for female tubal ligation.[9]

Female sterilisation is generally more invasive and carries higher risks compared to male sterilisation. Female sterilisation typically involves a laparoscopic procedure or mini-laparotomy, requiring general anaesthesia and resulting in a longer recovery time, with risks including infection and injury to internal organs. In contrast, male sterilisation (vasectomy) is less invasive, often performed under local anaesthesia with minimal incisions or even no scalpel techniques, leading to a shorter recovery period and fewer complications.

Both procedures are considered permanent, so careful consideration is necessary before choosing sterilisation. Reversal of tubal ligation is more complex and less successful than vasectomy reversal, and users who wish to conceive again are usually advised to opt for IVF rather than attempting to unblock the damaged fallopian tubes. Vasectomy reversal is possible, but it is not always successful, and the chances of restoring fertility decrease over time.

Can I ask for sterilisation if I have not had children and do not wish to in the future?

Yes, you can request sterilisation at a younger age if you are certain you do not wish to have children in the future. However, healthcare providers will typically conduct a thorough evaluation to ensure you fully understand the permanence of the procedure and are making an informed decision. They may discuss alternative contraception options and consider factors such as your age, health, and personal circumstances before proceeding. Also, sterilisation is just as effective at preventing pregnancy as other long-acting reversible contraception options which are less risky or invasive. It's important to have a detailed discussion with your provider about your decision and any potential implications.

Benefits of sterilisation

- **Highly effective:** Sterilisation is over 99% effective at preventing pregnancy, making it one of the most reliable contraceptive methods
- **Permanent solution:** It offers a long-term, permanent solution for those who are certain they do not want more children or have completed their family planning
- **Hormone free:** Sterilisation does not involve hormonal treatments, avoiding potential side effects associated with hormonal contraception

Risks of sterilisation

- **Permanent:** Sterilisation is intended to be permanent, and while reversals are possible, they are complex, not always successful, and may not restore fertility to previous levels
- **Surgical risks:** Both male and female sterilisation involve surgical procedures with associated risks, including infection, bleeding, and, in the case of female sterilisation, potential injury to internal organs
- **Potential for regret:** If life circumstances change and the desire for more children arises, the difficulty and uncertainty of reversal can lead to regret and emotional distress

Which contraceptive coil is right for me?

Contraceptive coils, or intrauterine devices (IUDs), are an excellent option for long-term birth control and managing menstrual symptoms. They come in two main types: non-hormonal copper IUDs and hormonal intrauterine systems (IUSs), like the Mirena or Jaydess. Both are highly effective but work differently, so choosing the right one depends on your needs and preferences.

Hormonal coil (IUS)

The IUS releases a small amount of progesterone hormone into the uterus, offering over 99% effectiveness in preventing pregnancy. It works by thickening cervical mucus to block sperm, thinning the womb lining to prevent implantation, and, in some cases, stopping ovulation. The hormonal coil is

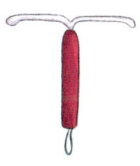

especially popular for managing heavy or painful periods, and many users experience lighter or even no periods after a year. It's also commonly used for non-contraceptive benefits, such as relieving PMS or protecting the womb lining during hormone replacement therapy (HRT).

Key benefits

- **Lighter or no periods**, with reduced period pain
- **Effective at preventing pregnancy** for up to 8 years (depending on which coil is used) and easy to reverse[10]
- **Lower hormone levels:** The IUS has the lowest level of hormone of all the hormonal methods of contraception. The hormones are focused in the womb rather than having generalised effects around your whole body. This can mean less side effects than other forms of contraception such as bloating or weight gain
- **Protects against endometrial cancer** by keeping the womb lining thin[11]

DID YOU KNOW?

You don't need to have a period once a month! The Mirena works by keeping the lining of the womb thin, so there is no need for a period. By 1 year after insertion, around 20% of people don't experience any bleeding at all (lucky them!). And 65% of users have either no bleeding, or reduced bleeding, after a year of using the hormonal coils.[12]

Potential drawbacks

- **Irregular bleeding**, particularly in the first few months
- **Some users report headaches**, mood changes, low libido, acne, or breast tenderness
- **Doesn't protect against STIs**; condoms may still be needed
- **Small risk of pelvic infection** if introduced during an untreated infection

Non-hormonal coil (copper IUD)

The copper IUD is hormone free and relies on copper to create an environment that prevents sperm survival and fertilisation. It's also over 99% effective, making it a great contraceptive option for those wanting to avoid hormones. The device can last 5–10 years, depending on the type. However, unlike the IUS, it doesn't reduce period symptoms and may initially cause heavier or more painful periods.

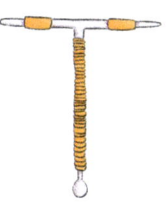

Key benefits

- **Hormone free**, so no risk of hormone-related side effects
- **Long-lasting** and immediately reversible upon removal
- **Ideal** for those concerned about long-term hormonal use

Hormonal coil – over 99% effective

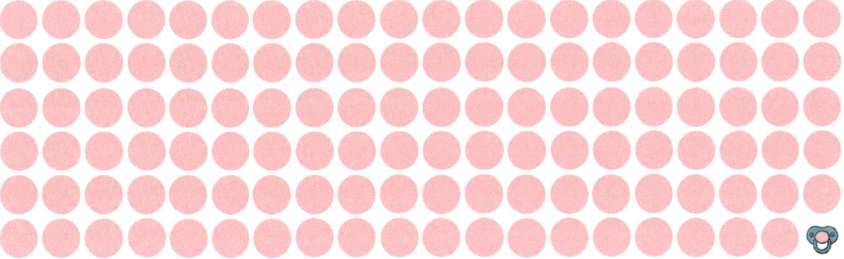

Copper coil – over 99% effective

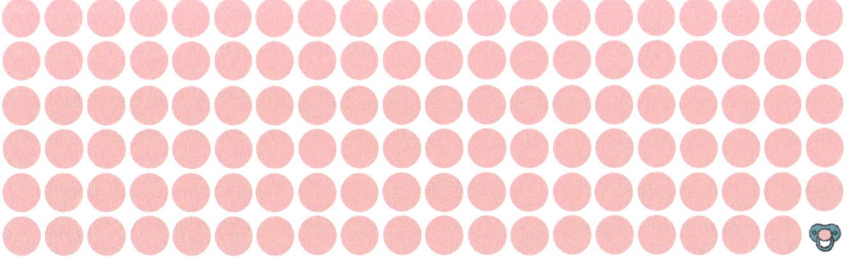

Potential drawbacks

- **May cause heavier** or longer periods initially
- **No protection** against STIs
- **Rare risk of pelvic infection** if fitted during an active infection

Choosing the right option

Your choice between the hormonal IUS and copper IUD depends on your priorities. If lighter periods and pain relief for periods are essential, the hormonal coil might be ideal. If you prefer a hormone-free option, the copper IUD is a reliable alternative. Discuss your preferences, medical history, and lifestyle with your doctor to make the best choice for your needs.

How are the coils inserted?

Both the IUD and IUS are put in by a doctor or nurse at a general practice surgery, sexual health clinic, or family planning clinic. They may also be inserted by a gynaecologist at the hospital during other procedures.

Before your IUD is fitted, the fitter will check inside your vagina for the position and size of your womb. You may be tested for any existing infections, such as STIs and for pregnancy.

The appointment takes about 20–30 minutes, and fitting the IUD should take no longer than 5 minutes:

- The vagina is held open using a speculum similar to a smear test
- Your cervix may be briefly held using a metal or plastic grasper which can sting
- The IUD is inserted through the cervix and into the womb

You may get period-type cramps afterwards, but painkillers can ease the cramps. You may also bleed for a few days after having an IUD fitted.

Once an IUD has been fitted, you can check for the thread position at 6 weeks to make sure everything is fine. Tell your general practitioner if you have any problems after this initial check or if you want the IUD removed. Sometimes a scan is arranged to confirm the position.

TOP TIPS FOR INSERTION AND REMOVAL:

 **CHOOSE THE RIGHT TIME:** Schedule the insertion for a time when you are not on your period. While it's possible to insert a coil during menstruation, if you have a very heavy flow, it may come out! A good time to consider is the last day or so of your period, as your cervix will still be open, but the flow will be light

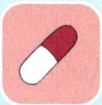 **TAKE PAIN RELIEF BEFOREHAND:** Consider taking an over-the-counter pain reliever (such as ibuprofen) before the procedure to help manage any discomfort

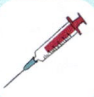 **DISCUSS ANAESTHESIA OPTIONS:** If you are anxious or concerned about pain, discuss anaesthesia options with your healthcare provider. Some providers may offer local anaesthesia to numb the cervix

 **BRING A SUPPORT PERSON:** Having a friend or family member accompany you to the appointment can provide emotional support and assistance with transportation, especially if you feel anxious

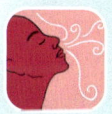 **PRACTICE RELAXATION TECHNIQUES:** Practice deep breathing or other relaxation techniques to help manage anxiety before and during the procedure. Inform your healthcare provider if you have concerns or fears or if you suffer from vaginismus

 **WEAR COMFORTABLE CLOTHING:** Wear loose and comfortable clothing to the appointment to help you feel more at ease during the procedure and just after

Coil FAQs

How soon does it work to prevent pregnancy?

- Copper coil (IUD) – immediate
- Mirena/Jaydess (IUS) fitted before day 5 of menstrual cycle – immediate
- Mirena/Jaydess (IUS) fitted after day 5 of menstrual cycle – 7 days after insertion

They can be taken out very easily by a doctor or nurse whenever you decide you no longer want the device or wish to conceive.

Is it right for my lifestyle?

Coils are a fantastic option for people with busy lives or those who prefer a low-maintenance contraceptive method. Once inserted, they last between 5 and 10 years, depending on the type, and don't require daily attention like the pill. They're also not affected by other medications, or issues like vomiting or diarrhoea, making them a reliable option regardless of your health or routine.

Will my partner feel the coil during sex?

In some cases, partners may feel the threads of the coil during sex. These threads are soft but can be trimmed by a healthcare professional if they are noticeable or cause discomfort. Over time, the threads often soften further and become less noticeable.

When can it be used after birth?

In some cases, an IUD/IUS can be fitted within 48 hours of giving birth so you can request this prior to delivery so your healthcare team are prepared. Otherwise, the IUD or IUS can usually be fitted 4 weeks after giving birth (vaginal or caesarean). You'll need to use alternative contraception from 3 weeks (21 days) after the birth until the IUD/IUS is put in. It's safe to use an IUD/IUS when you're breastfeeding, and it will not affect your milk supply.

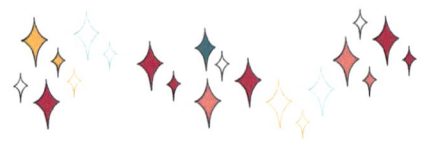

Breastfeeding and contraception

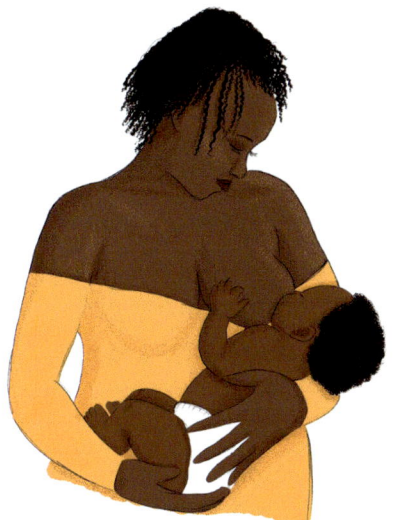

You can actually get pregnant as early as 21 days after birth. Breastfeeding can be used as a form of contraception (lactational amenorrhoea method, described above) but it is not 100% effective at preventing conception, and lots of factors need to be carefully controlled or it can fail, leading to pregnancy.

There are other excellent options for contraception while breastfeeding:

- A coil (IUD or IUS) can be fitted, either within 48 hours of giving birth, or from 4 weeks postpartum which will give a long-acting, reliable form of contraception

- The POP, depot injection, progesterone implant or, of course, condoms can all be used reliably from any time after birth

- From 3 weeks after birth when formula feeding, or 6 weeks after birth if breastfeeding, you can start the combined hormonal contraception (CHC) options (the pill or the patch)

There is no evidence that progesterone in contraception affects milk supply, but anecdotally some women report that it does. Oestrogen-containing contraceptives may have more of an effect on milk production, so some people prefer to avoid these forms of contraception while breastfeeding.

Will my contraception affect fertility later?

A common concern about hormonal contraception is whether it impacts long-term fertility. The good news is that hormonal contraceptives – such as pills, patches, injections, and intrauterine systems – prevent pregnancy temporarily by suppressing ovulation, thickening cervical mucus, and altering the uterine lining. Once you stop using them, these effects reverse, and, for most people, ovulation resumes within a few weeks to months.

Key points to bear in mind:

- **Return to fertility can be slow:** Most individuals regain normal fertility quickly after stopping hormonal contraception, with ovulation typically resuming within 3 months. Long-acting methods like the injection may take slightly longer to wear off, but fertility eventually returns to baseline

- **Age-related fertility:** Fertility naturally declines with age, particularly after 35. This decline is unrelated to past contraceptive use. If you start contraception earlier in life, it may mask underlying fertility issues, such as polycystic ovary syndrome (PCOS) or endometriosis, that only become apparent after stopping

- **Underlying health conditions:** Hormonal contraceptives can manage symptoms of conditions like endometriosis or irregular cycles. When discontinued, these conditions may resurface, potentially affecting fertility. However, this is due to the condition itself, not the contraception

If you are taking contraception but thinking about conceiving in the near future, it's helpful to discuss this with your doctor, who can provide guidance on when to stop contraception and assess any fertility-related concerns early.

Emergency contraception (the morning-after pill)

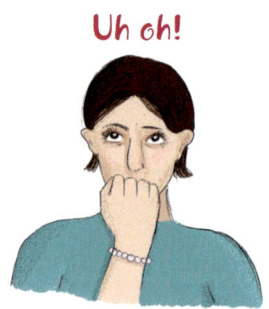

Uh oh!

The morning-after pill is rarely discussed in popular culture, and unfortunately – like many subjects that involve the female body – is still shrouded in stigma. This makes it a difficult topic to bring up, and therefore a difficult subject to find information on.

You probably know it as the 'morning-after pill', but a more accurate name is emergency contraception, which is used to avoid the misconception that it can only be administered the morning after sexual intercourse.

In fact, both pill options available in the UK (and the IUD option) can be effective even 3–5 days after sex, although keep in mind that it's one of those ASAP situations.

We also call it 'emergency' contraception to make it clear that this shouldn't be a regular option that you rely on. Yes, it's nice to know its available in the back of your mind, but it's not as reliable at preventing pregnancy as contraception that is taken on a regular basis, so if you are certain about wanting to avoid an unplanned pregnancy, there are better options out there for you!

Why does stigma exist?

There has long been a silence around this much-needed medicine. Perhaps sometimes it's unjustified embarrassment over having had unprotected sex (things happen, it's nothing to be ashamed of!), and sometimes it's due to the misconception that taking the morning-after pill causes an abortion (it doesn't).

No one should ever feel this stigma in the modern world we live in, but it is understandable that you may not want to walk into a pharmacy shouting you want emergency contraception at the top of your voice. You can always ask for the medications by their formal brand name or ask to talk to a pharmacist privately. Either way, it's best to be informed about your options, so let's dive in …

Who can take emergency contraception?

Most women and people who have periods can use it, even those who can't use hormonal contraception. There are a few caveats to that, so if you have allergies to any of its ingredients, a history of asthma, or are taking other medications, discuss this with your doctor first.

What does it do?

Emergency contraception works by delaying or preventing ovulation, making it most effective when taken as soon as possible after unprotected sex.

There are two main types: levonorgestrel pills (Plan B, Levonelle), which are 98% effective and work up to 72 hours (sometimes 120 hours) after sex, and ulipristal acetate (ellaOne), which is 99% effective for up to 120 hours.

Depending on the egg's progress, these pills either prevent sperm from fertilising your eggs, temporarily stop the release of an egg from your ovary or prevent fertilised eggs from implanting in the uterus. It's really very clever! However, it is important to be completely clear; they do NOT cause abortion because no pregnancy has ever implanted in the womb.

Keep in mind though that if you have already ovulated, the emergency contraception pill will much less effective at preventing a pregnancy from implanting so it's even more important to go for regular contraception rather than emergency contraception if you can avoid it!

When can you take it?

It is always best to take emergency contraception as soon as possible, because the sooner you take it, the more options you have – some must be taken within 72 hours, and others can be taken up to 120 hours from unprotected intercourse. Remember that the longer it has been, the less effective the emergency contraception will be!

An IUD can also be used as a form of emergency contraception, and this can be fitted up to 5 days after having unprotected sex, in order to be effective, and then has the added bonus of providing you with reliable contraception longer term. If inserted on time, less than 1% of women who use one will get pregnant.

What about side effects?

Luckily, there aren't any serious side effects of taking emergency contraception, but it can bring on headaches or even stomach pain and could make you feel nauseous or vomit. If you are sick within 2 hours of taking Levonelle, or 3 hours of taking ellaOne, be sure to see your healthcare provider or pharmacist ASAP to take another dose. You may also notice that it messes up your cycle slightly, as your next period may be on time, early or late. If your period is over a week late make sure you do a pregnancy test to be sure.

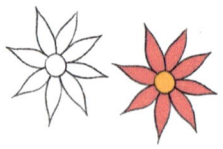

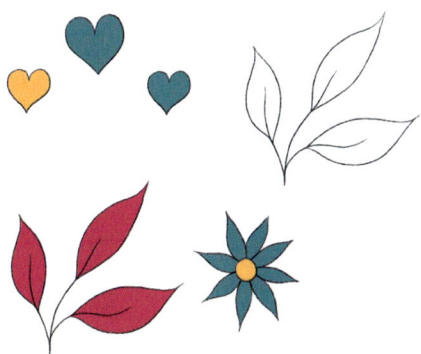

So, there you have it: we've explored a range of contraception options, each with its unique benefits, mechanisms, and considerations. From hormonal methods like the IUS and various types of IUDs to hormone-free choices and emergency contraception, it's clear that choosing the right method involves weighing up factors such as how it is taken, side effects, and personal preferences. Even with this deep dive we have just scratched the surface about what there is to say about contraception!

The most important thing is to weigh up what makes the perfect contraception for you and discuss your main goals with your healthcare professional to find the best choice.

Bumps come in all shapes and sizes

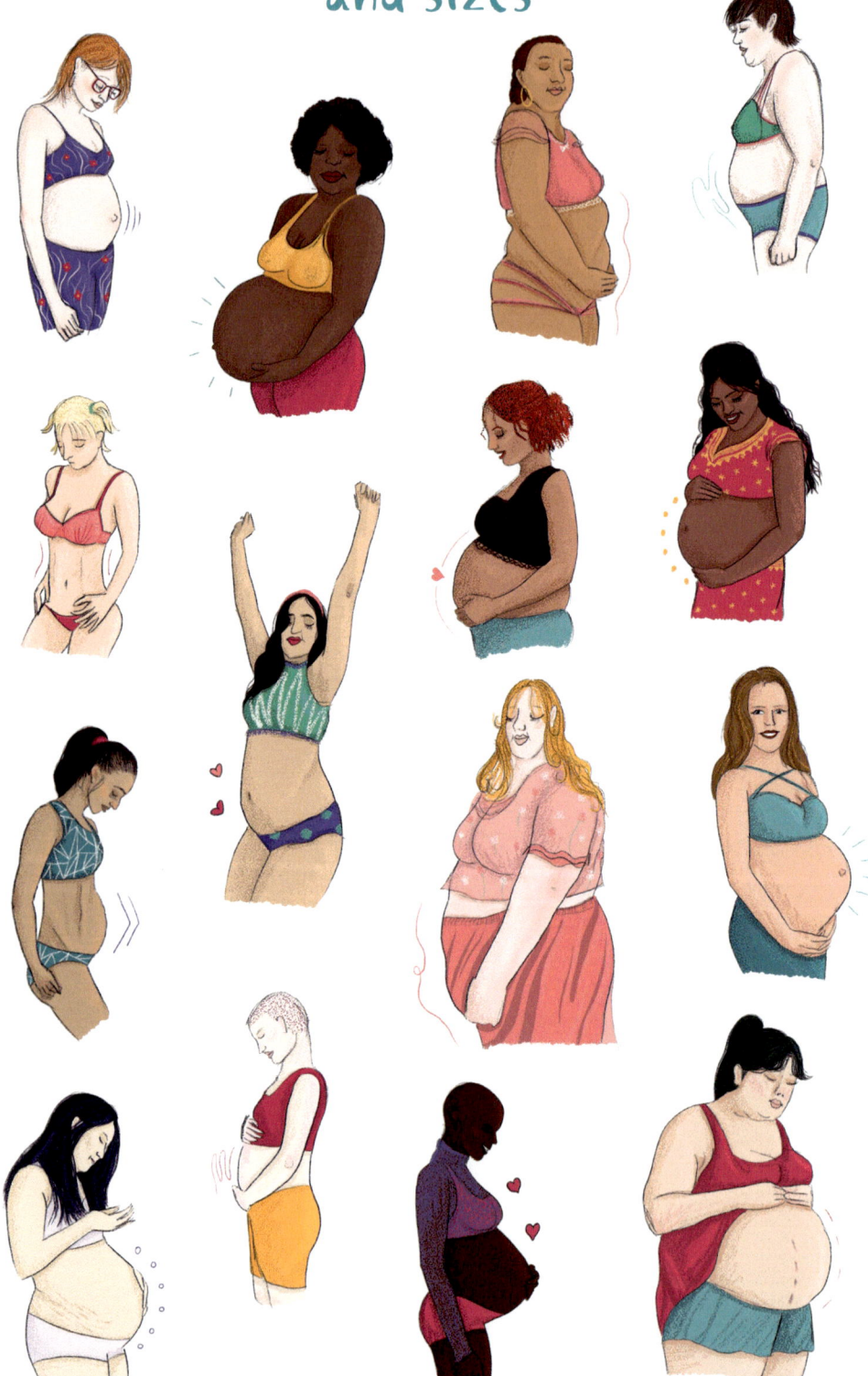

CHAPTER 7

Pregnancy

What should you do when you find out you are pregnant?

Discovering that you are pregnant is a momentous occasion, brimming with a spectrum of emotions ranging from excitement and joy to apprehension, uncertainty, or even sadness. In this chapter, we'll explore key tips and facts about pregnancy, as well as some helpful guidance to manage your ever-changing body.

Navigating the first steps

Initial reactions

There is no right way to react when you find out you are pregnant. First off, just breathe. There's nothing that you need to do immediately. Take it all in and think about what this moment means for you. How do you feel? Are you happy or are you sad? Do you need to tell your partner? Do you want to tell anybody else?

Traditionally, people often avoid telling friends and family until their 12-week scan. There are many reasons you may choose to do this; the risk of miscarriage is highest in the first trimester so people commonly wish to wait until they are certain the pregnancy will progress. The first trimester can be a time filled with fear and anxiety so it might be something you prefer to deal with on your own, keeping the news to yourself until you can relax, when the risk of miscarriage reduces, typically after 12 weeks. However, there isn't any reason you can't tell people sooner if you want to! Especially if you feel like you would benefit from the support of your loved ones.

Calculating your due date

Before you get in touch with the hospital it is helpful to work out how far along your pregnancy is. You will need your period dates; identify the first day of your last period, and you can then input this into any online due-date calculator. This will calculate an estimated due date, and also estimate how many weeks pregnant you are. If you weren't keeping track of your periods, you can let the midwife know that you aren't sure when your estimated due date will be, and they may recommend an earlier pregnancy scan. These figures are just a guide; it is important to know that your due date will later be confirmed at your 10–12-week scan.

Contacting healthcare providers

One of the first steps after confirming your pregnancy is to contact your healthcare provider. They will guide you through the next steps, begin prenatal care by addressing any existing medical conditions or medications you take, and answering any questions or concerns you may have. There is no rush to do this immediately if you have found out about your pregnancy very early, but you should aim to have your first appointment by around 8–9 weeks of pregnancy. Depending on healthcare practices in your region, you may be advised to schedule an initial prenatal appointment within the first few weeks of pregnancy.

DID YOU KNOW?

The first pregnancy scan is typically around 12 weeks, and serves several purposes. It confirms the pregnancy is viable by checking that the fetus has developed visible features like limbs and a head. The scan is used to accurately determine the baby's age, helping to predict a reliable due date and monitor growth milestones. Additionally, the scan may include a measurement known as the nuchal translucency (NT) test. Combining the NT measurement with maternal age and other factors can determine if further tests should be offered to assess the risk of chromosomal conditions like Down syndrome.

So, while it seems a bit mean to be told to wait until 10–12 weeks to have your first scan, there is good reason for this. Scanning earlier in the pregnancy wouldn't be able to assess if the fetus has developed as expected. It can also provide false reassurance about the pregnancy because, unfortunately, it is possible to see a heartbeat and a normal looking fetus initially, but later miscarry the pregnancy.

If you experience any bleeding or pain in pregnancy, you should always seek help from a healthcare professional, and you may be offered an earlier scan to check for the possibility of miscarriage or ectopic pregnancy.

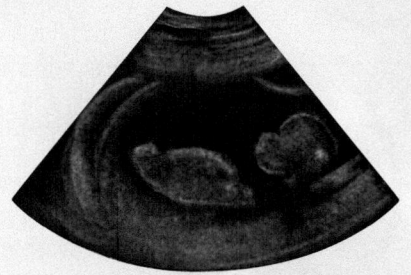

TOP TIPS FOR THE FIRST TRIMESTER:

The first trimester of pregnancy is considered to begin on the first day of your period and continue until the end of week 12. It involves many changes happening at the same time, from the intense physical changes, a rollercoaster of emotions, and a list of practicalities to consider.

Here are some top tips for changes you can make in order to optimise the pregnancy and to help you manage the challenges the first trimester brings!

 ## LIFESTYLE CHANGES

You may have been planning your pregnancy for a while, and already made a lot of changes. However, if you haven't, now is the time to cut out alcohol, smoking, and any other medications or drugs that are not pregnancy-safe. Even if this pregnancy was unexpected for you, and you're undecided about continuing, these changes are worth making until you decide.

Prioritise rest, as fatigue is common, especially if you have other children. Adjust your plans, ask for help with childcare, or just accept that the children may have a bit more screen-time than you would like to get you through this particularly challenging stretch!

If you are working, and you feel comfortable, speak to your employer about what adjustments may make this time easier, such as adjusting your working hours or the option to sometimes work from home.

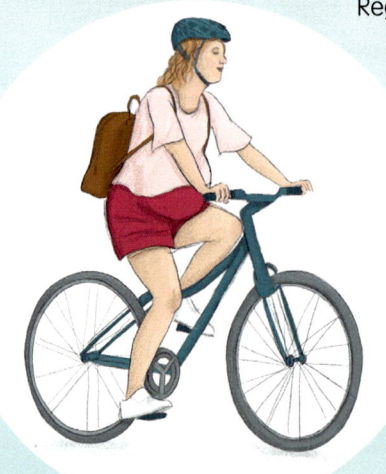

Regular exercise is great for both your pregnancy and your mental well-being. You may have to adjust your normal routine as your symptoms allow and take a gentler approach for a few weeks. However, you can rest assured that exercise is safe in early pregnancy.

Adjust your caffeine intake; ideally, you want to restrict your caffeine intake to about 200 milligrams a day. This generally means one latte and then swap out the rest of your drinks for a decaffeinated alternative.

continued...

What does 200 mg of caffeine look like?

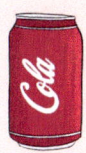 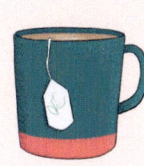 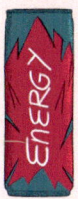

Can of cola + mug of tea + 250 ml can energy drink = **195 mg caffeine**

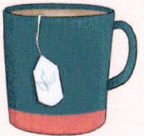 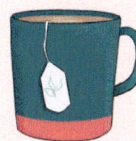 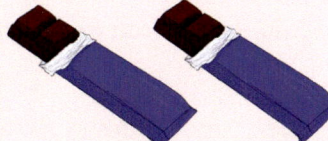

Mug of tea + mug of tea + small bar of dark chocolate + small bar of dark chocolate = **200 mg caffeine**

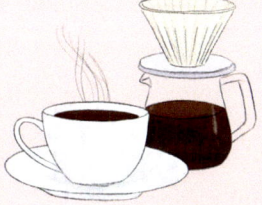 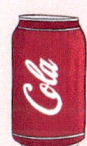

Cup of filter coffee + can of cola = **180 mg caffeine**

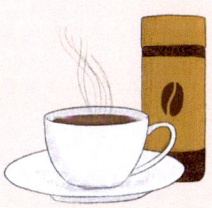 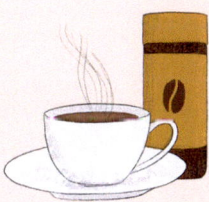

Cup of instant coffee + cup of instant coffee = **200 mg caffeine**

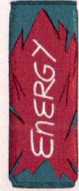 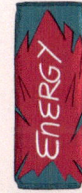 

250ml can energy drink + 250ml can energy drink + can of cola = **200 mg caffeine**

Focus on maintaining a balanced diet, which is rich in fresh fruit and vegetables, and also stay hydrated. Certain foods should be avoided due to the risk of infections that can be transmitted to the baby. Exactly what you should avoid may depend on where you are in the world but typically during pregnancy you should avoid raw fish, unpasteurised cheeses and liver, or other such foods containing vitamin A.

 ## REVIEW YOUR MEDICATIONS

If you take regular medications, check with your doctor to ensure they are safe for pregnancy. In the meantime, you can also check the safety of medications on another great resource: the Bumps website.[1] This is better than reading the back of the medication packets, which may say to avoid in pregnancy, but there is more nuance to this. Some medications, like paracetamol, are fine, while others, such as certain blood pressure medications, may need adjusting. You should never stop medications, like antidepressants, suddenly without medical advice as your doctor can guide you on whether to continue, change, or wean off safely.

For supplements, folic acid and vitamin D are essential in early pregnancy, and iron may be recommended later, based on blood tests. Many multivitamins are available, which contain these vitamins as well as a variety of others.

👍 **Money saving hack:** Most supermarkets and pharmacies sell cheaper versions of certain vitamin supplements, and as long as they contain the recommended 400 micrograms of folic acid, they are absolutely sufficient!

 ## SEEK SUPPORT

The first trimester often comes with additional challenges, especially if you experience symptoms like nausea, vomiting, and exhaustion. You should feel comfortable to speak to your doctor for advice on ways to manage these symptoms, but you should also be encouraged to lean on your support network for emotional support and practical assistance.

The risk of miscarriage is highest in the first trimester, although this risk decreases as the trimester progresses. Therefore, this can be a very anxious time especially if you have been through previous losses or fertility struggles. Reaching out to a trusted friend can help to talk through those worries.

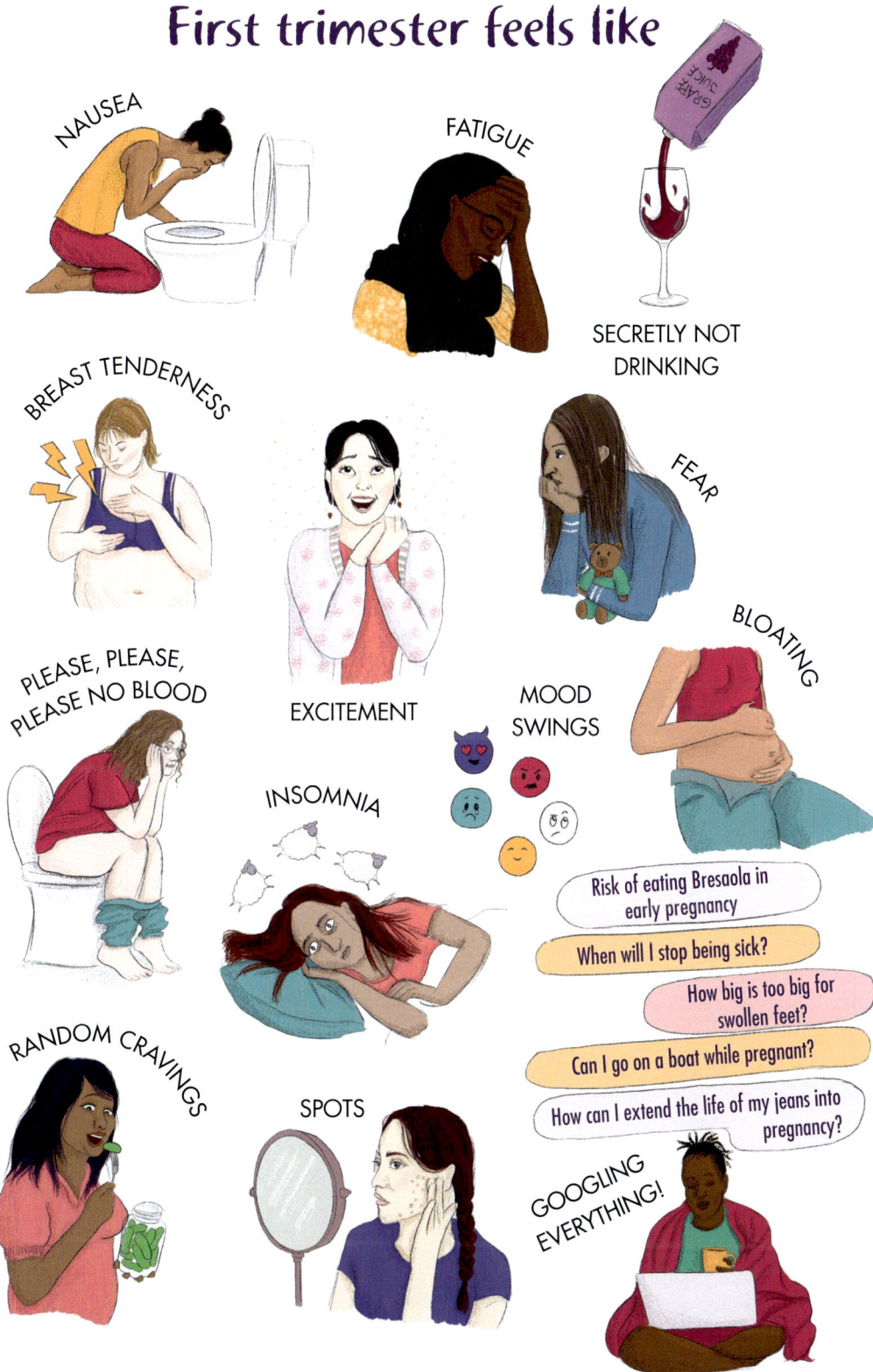

Tips for surviving pregnancy nausea

For too long we have suffered in silence! There are so many options to help pregnancy sickness, rather than just getting on with it and accepting it as part of life.

Nausea and vomiting in pregnancy (NVP) is a common condition affecting approximately 70% of pregnant women. It is misleadingly referred to as 'morning sickness'. Only 1.8% of women report morning-only symptoms, whereas 80% report all-day nausea![2]

A more severe form of NVP is a condition called hyperemesis gravidarum (HG), which affects approximately 1–1.5% of pregnancies. The main difference between HG and typical NVP is that the nausea and vomiting is so severe that you are unable to eat and/or drink normally and daily activities become almost impossible. It can result in weight loss and severe dehydration, sometimes requiring admission to hospital for treatment.

For the majority of people, the sickness improves around 12–14 weeks but for others it can persist until 20 weeks or beyond.

TOP TIPS FOR PREGNANCY NAUSEA:

 1. **EXPERIMENT WITH FLUIDS:** Try juices, ice chips, using a straw, or thicker options like milkshakes or smoothies

 2. **EAT SMALL MEALS:** Try small, frequent meals or snacks throughout the day

 3. **KEEP IT SIMPLE:** Opt for bland, salty, or high-protein foods that are easier to tolerate

 4. **AVOID STRONG COOKING SMELLS:** Focus on pre-prepared or cold foods

 5. **CONSIDER WORKPLACE ADJUSTMENTS:** Ask about flexible hours or remote work, if nausea affects your routine

 6. **PREPARE A 'NAUSEA KIT' FOR OUTINGS:** Take water, hard candies, wipes, and a sick bag (nappy sacks work well)

Remember, anti-sickness medications are safe and can be helpful if needed to prevent dehydration or severe symptoms.

Myth   **It only happens in the morning**

Fact   Nope! Morning sickness can hit at any time of day, and many people may find, in fact, that it worsens in the evening!

Myth   **Everyone gets pregnancy cravings**

Fact   Another misconception: some people find themselves experiencing strong cravings, or even food aversions but others don't notice any changes at all!

Myth   **Baby can still grow even if you can't keep anything down**

Fact   This is actually true: your baby gets the nutrients before you do, so even if you are starving, losing weight, and becoming dehydrated, your baby is usually still able to grow. However, in severe cases of hyperemesis it is important to keep an eye on the growth of the baby with regular scans to be sure.

Myth   **You just have to put up with the nausea and vomiting**

Fact   This is completely false. There are many effective anti-sickness medications (anti-emetics) that have been extensively used in pregnancy for decades, and are considered safe by major health organisations. Untreated severe nausea or hyperemesis gravidarum (HG) can lead to serious complications, so it's considered better to take these well-established treatments if needed. You don't have to endure debilitating symptoms – help is available, and it's safe to seek relief for the sake of both you and your baby.

What to expect from the second trimester

The second trimester of your pregnancy spans week 13 to week 28 (months 4–6). For many, this part of pregnancy can bring some relief; symptoms begin to ease and the risk of miscarriage drops, meaning you can start to relax and you are likely to feel an increase in your general energy levels.

As you go through the second trimester, you'll gradually see your 'bump' grow and later you'll start to feel your baby moving.

THESE THINGS ARE TOTALLY NORMAL!

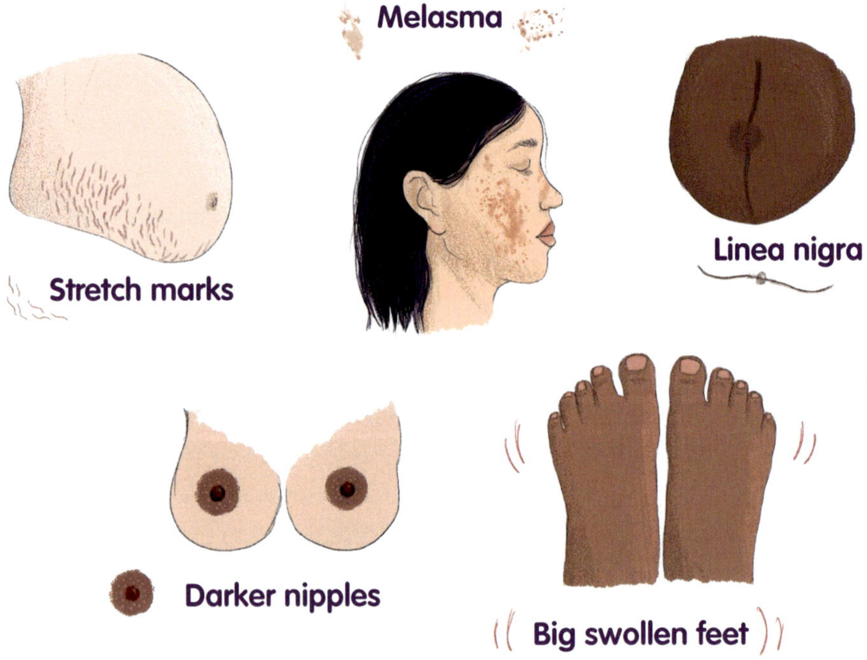

Melasma

Stretch marks

Linea nigra

Darker nipples

Big swollen feet

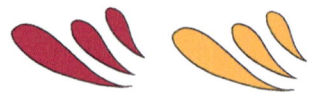

When will I feel my baby move?

For first-time pregnancies, you might feel your baby move – often called 'quickening' – between 18 and 23 weeks, though this varies. Movements can feel like flutters or gas at first and become more distinctly recognisable as kicks, flutters, or rolls as the baby grows. Women who have been pregnant before may feel these movements a bit earlier because they are more attuned to the sensations.

Several factors influence timing: an anterior placenta (front of the uterus) may cushion movements. However, once you start to feel them, you should continue to feel them regularly, so it isn't a reason to ignore a change in baby's movements or dismiss it as being due to an anterior placenta! People with higher body mass indexes (BMIs) might also take longer to feel fetal movements because the extra layers of tissue can dampen the sensation. By 28 weeks, you should notice a regular pattern of movements.

While variations in the timing of fetal movements are normal, sudden changes to the pattern or a lack of movement should be discussed with a healthcare professional. Never ignore it and trust your gut!

Top tips for your second trimester

Book your anatomy scan

Your second ultrasound scan will usually be scheduled around 20 weeks of pregnancy. This is often described as the anatomy scan, because it aims to check all the parts of the fetus's anatomy: the baby's bones, heart, brain, spinal cord, face, kidneys, and abdomen. This scan is also the opportunity to find out the baby's sex if you wish. Some parents are excited to find out and others prefer to be surprised at the birth. Keep in mind, though, that it isn't always possible to determine the gender with certainty, as it can depend on the position of baby, and is not always 100% accurate.

You have the right to say no to any test or scan that's offered. It is always your choice and the team looking after you should respect your decisions.

Consider your options for place of birth

If you haven't already thought about it, it's a good time to start thinking about where and how you would like to have your baby. Depending on where you live and your medical history, you may have the option to choose an alternative to a hospital birth, potentially planning to use a birth centre or have a home birth. You can discuss the pros and cons of these options with your midwife.

Exercise

Staying active during pregnancy benefits both you and your baby. By staying fit and active in your second trimester, you can prepare your body for the challenges of labour as well as the physical challenges of being a new parent! If you had to reduce your activity during the first trimester, then the second trimester is a great time to get back into it while you have some energy.

Focus on activities you enjoy, like walking, swimming, or gentle yoga, and don't stress about intensity or hitting the usual number of reps. Manage your expectations while you are growing another human, and remember that just moving your body in any way is a healthy and positive step forward!

Tips for safe pregnancy exercise

- **Safe options:** walking, swimming, stationary cycling, modified yoga/Pilates, or light strength training
- **Avoid:** exercises that involve lying flat after 16 weeks, rapid twists and turns and changes of direction that may cause joint damage, contact sports, activities with a high risk of falls, and overheating (e.g., hot yoga)
- **Cautions:** Use proper technique for weightlifting and avoid heavy barbells or focused core exercises after 12 weeks

Benefits of staying active[3]

- It boosts energy, reduces stress and anxiety, and improves sleep
- It helps manage healthy weight gain and postpartum body positivity
- It can improve side effects such as constipation and reduces the risk of complications like gestational diabetes or preeclampsia
- It may shorten labour and improve overall delivery outcomes
- There is also a suggestion that brain development in the baby may be boosted by regular exercise during pregnancy[4]

If you have always been active, continuing to exercise at the same level when pregnant is safe and healthy.

If you need something to build up to here are the recommendations:

 strength exercises on two or more days a week that work all the major muscle groups

 75 minutes of vigorous activity a week OR

 150 minutes of moderate activity

Always listen to your body and consult your healthcare provider for personalised advice.

The third trimester – getting ready!

The third trimester specifically refers to weeks 28 until birth (usually up to 42 weeks gestation). The final weeks of pregnancy can be more challenging as the weight of the growing baby becomes more of an effort to carry. Then you add tiredness, sore and painful joints, difficulty getting a good night's sleep, and that pressure of the baby on your cervix! Even just rolling over can feel like doing a difficult three-point turn!

It can feel quite overwhelming to wrap your mind around the birth, and also the impending arrival and all the changes that will bring.

Here is my ultimate guide to what you can do in the final weeks to give yourself the best chance of staying comfortable and active until the end of pregnancy.

Staying active and managing pain

As the end of pregnancy approaches, your growing bump can make exercising awkward and carrying the extra weight can be tiring. In the third trimester you can carry on exercising as long as you feel well and comfortable. If you feel okay, you can stay active right up to the birth of your baby.

If you are experiencing pelvic pain, ask for a referral to see a women's health physiotherapist who can give you some ideas and specific focused exercises to help improve the pain.

Do babies run out of room during pregnancy?

As your baby grows during the course of your pregnancy, it can definitely feel like you are running out of space. There is a common misconception that babies may move less towards the end of pregnancy because there is less room for them to move around, but it is important to clear this myth up.

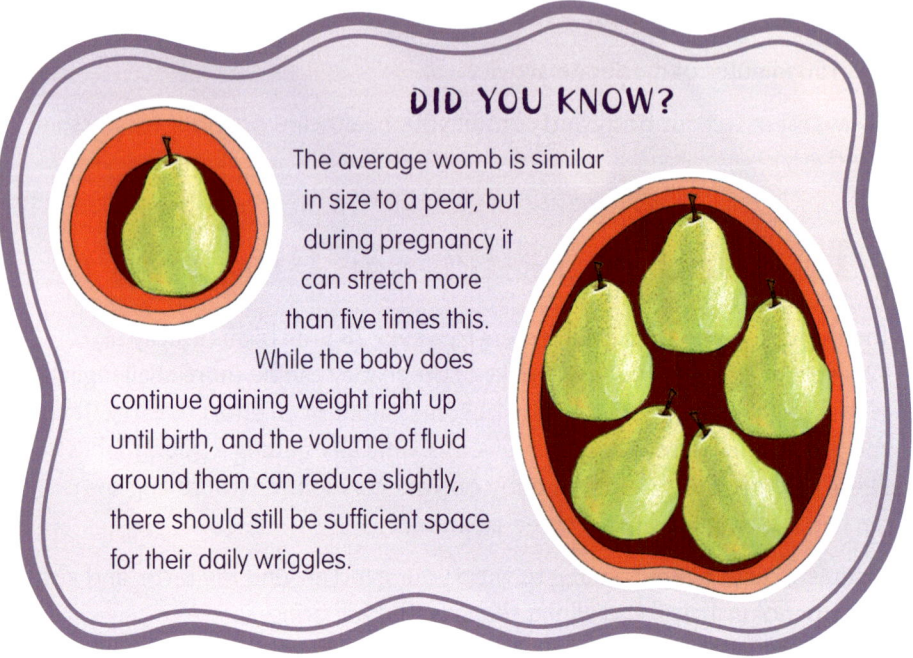

DID YOU KNOW?

The average womb is similar in size to a pear, but during pregnancy it can stretch more than five times this. While the baby does continue gaining weight right up until birth, and the volume of fluid around them can reduce slightly, there should still be sufficient space for their daily wriggles.

What can you expect from your movements?

Most people will first feel their baby move at between 16 and 24 weeks, generally increasing up to around 32 weeks. In the later part of your third trimester, the type of movements felt may differ, but you should continue to feel baby move up to and during labour.

If your baby's movements seem noticeably reduced, you should contact your midwife so they can listen to baby's heartbeat or arrange a scan. You wouldn't normally be expected to have a pattern to the movements until after 28 weeks, and after this time point it is important to monitor how often you feel the movements, and when, so you can be aware if there is any significant change from usual.

Every baby has its own 'normal' regarding frequency of movement. However, if you ever feel your baby is moving significantly less than their normal, please don't hesitate to contact your maternity team – as often as you need to!

Can you have sex during pregnancy?

Yes, you can have sex during pregnancy, unless your healthcare provider advises otherwise. For most pregnancies, sex is completely safe and won't harm the baby, who is well protected by the amniotic sac and the uterus. Hormonal changes during pregnancy may even increase sexual desire for some, though others might feel less interested due to fatigue, nausea, or other symptoms. The key is to communicate openly with your partner and explore comfortable positions as your body changes.

However, certain conditions might require caution, such as a low-lying placenta (placenta previa), cervical insufficiency, or if you've been advised to avoid sex due to bleeding or preterm labour risk. If you have any concerns or experience unusual symptoms like pain or spotting after sex, consult your healthcare provider. Pregnancy is a time of change, so focus on what feels right for you and your relationship.

Other ideas to prepare for the birth of your baby

- Sign up for antenatal classes to prepare for every stage of labour and delivery; I recommend attending these with your birth partner so they are also prepped for what to expect!

- Consider learning about hypnobirthing – this is a series of techniques that include breathing methods and mindfulness, which have been proven to reduce the need for pain relief medication during labour and improve overall experience of birth

- Practice perineal massage to lower the risk of severe tearing or needing an episiotomy as your baby's head stretches your perineum during birth

PERINEAL MASSAGE GUIDE

Start after 35 weeks. Try to do this 1–2 times a week.

STEP 1

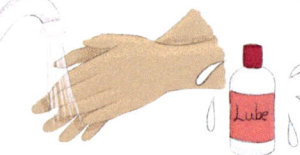

Wash your hands and then lubricate the vulva, vaginal opening, and your thumb. Dip your fingers in lubricant

Find a comfy spot reclining in a bath or on your bed.

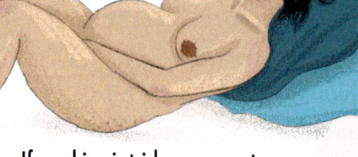

If reaching is tricky, your partner can help too!

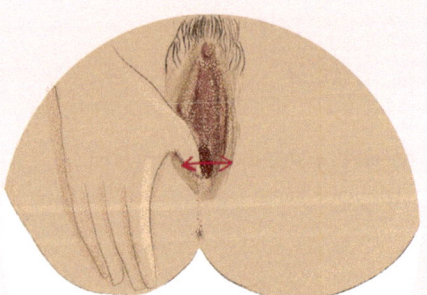

STEP 2 Place your thumb approximately one inch inside the vagina and sweep side to side, 10 times

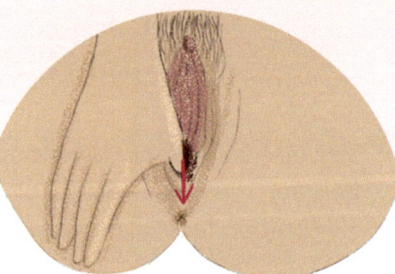

STEP 3 Hold and stretch towards your anus at the 6 o'clock position for 30 seconds. Then repeat this in all directions from 3 to 9 o'clock

196

TOP TIPS FOR LABOUR AND BIRTH:

 PACK YOUR HOSPITAL BAG: Include essentials for yourself and your baby, and keep your baby's first nappy and outfit in a separate bag for quick access

 GET AS MUCH SLEEP AS YOU CAN: Much easier said than done! A pregnancy pillow can give some extra support if you feel uncomfortable from the growing bump and changing joints

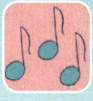 **PREPARE YOUR BIRTH SPACE:** Think about what you would like to see, smell, hear, and feel. That might include a particular music playlist, positive affirmations you can put up on the walls, a fan, or maybe a cold compress for your forehead

 KEEP MOVING: Buy an exercise ball so that even while at home watching TV you can bounce and move and encourage your contractions to build

 CALL AHEAD BEFORE HEADING TO THE HOSPITAL: They can help you to work out the best time to come in when your labour is progressing

What happens in labour?

 Labour is the process which ultimately leads to the birth of your baby. It usually begins between 37 and 42 weeks of pregnancy, but it can happen earlier than this, in which case it would be known as 'preterm labour'. It can be a very exciting time, but also can feel very uncertain and overwhelming.

A particularly helpful tip is to stay positive and keep an open mind. Focus on the parts of the process that are within your control, and let go of those that aren't. For example, whether you have a caesarean section or not depends on many factors, such as your contractions and the position and size of your baby. While you may not be able to change these things yourself, instead you can focus on trying to optimise the frequency and strength of your contractions by staying mobile, staying hydrated, and also by using breathing techniques to stay calm and lower your adrenaline.

How do I know if I am in labour?

1. **The 'show':** This is the mucus plug that sits within the cervix during pregnancy. As the cervix softens and opens, the mucus plug can be released and appear as discharge in your underwear. It may be clear or brownish and may even have slight streaks of blood in it. It is not actually a sign of labour but it can be a positive sign of changes that are happening, as it can be released days or even weeks before labour actually begins. Some women notice it after a membrane sweep or once labour has already started. Others may never see it at all!

2. **Contractions:** These are tightenings of the uterus, where your bump feels like it hardens and then relaxes again. The difference between contractions and Braxton Hicks is that contractions are more uncomfortable, as they can feel more like a period cramp and may build from your back round to your abdomen. They usually build in their intensity and frequency as labour progresses. A sign that you have entered the active phase of labour is that the contractions are coming every 3–5 minutes regularly, and they are lasting 60–90 seconds at a time

3. **Waters releasing:** When your waters break, this may be felt as a full-on gush, where a large volume of clear fluid comes out at once. Alternatively, you may instead have a trickle of a small amount of fluid. If you think your waters have broken, put on a sanitary towel, note the time, and look at the colour. The water around your baby should be clear or pinkish in colour. This process can happen before labour, or it may occur once labour has already commenced. Some babies are even born with the sac of waters still intact. If you think your waters have broken, let your midwife or your hospital know

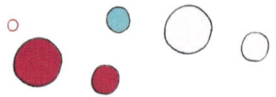

Braxton Hicks vs Contractions
What is the difference?

Don't represent active labour and can start at any point in pregnancy

Part of active labour

Regular, usually get closer together as labour progresses

Irregular and unpredictable, may come frequently and then taper or stop altogether

Last 60–90 seconds with a peak in the middle

Last anywhere from 15 seconds to 5 minutes

Continue despite movement or resting

Can occur in response to moving, walking or changing position

Get progressively more uncomfortable or painful

Not painful, although the squeezing sensation may be uncomfortable

May start from the back and spread around the front

The phases of labour

Early labour (latent phase)

This is the first stage of labour, where contractions start, but they are usually mild and irregular. During this phase, the cervix begins to soften, thin (efface), and open (dilate) up to 4 cm.

The tricky thing about this latent phase of labour is that it is very unpredictable. It means that you can start to have contractions but then they die off again, and this start/stop process can last for several hours or even days for some women. Some women may not notice these early contractions at all. If your contractions are not yet regular, you will be encouraged to stay at home, rest, and stay active, by walking or using a birthing ball, to help things to progress.

199

First stage of active labour

You will know you have entered the next phase of labour when the contractions become regular, and they begin to increase in intensity. This phase is characterised by more intense and regular contractions, typically lasting around 60–90 seconds and occurring every 3–5 minutes.

This stage takes your cervix from around 3–4 cm to fully dilated (10 cm). During this time, you will be experiencing regular contractions, and the intensity will increase so you may need to use breathing and relaxation techniques to cope with contractions. You can also opt for any form of pain relief you wish during this time.

Second stage – the birthing phase

Once you reach fully dilated, your baby's head is ready to be pushed down into the vagina for delivery. Women may experience a range of intense sensations, including pressure in the pelvic area, nausea, shaking, and hot flushes as they reach this point.

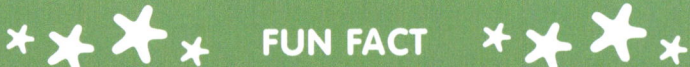 FUN FACT

Transition in the second stage of labour is a critical phase where the body shifts from the first stage to the second stage and the baby's head drops lower into the pelvis. It is often characterised by intense, frequent contractions, and can be emotionally and physically challenging as it is accompanied by a sudden adrenaline surge. During this time, many women experience strong feelings of self-doubt and may express sentiments like 'I can't do it anymore.' Or they even say things like 'I want to go home'.

These feelings are a normal part of labour and indicate that birth is imminent. The transition phase is typically the most intense, but it is also the shortest part of labour. This phase ends when the cervix is fully dilated, and the baby begins to move down the birth canal, signalling the start of the pushing stage.

When you first reach 10 cm, your medical team will sometimes encourage you to wait some time, up to 2 hours, to allow the contractions to bring the baby's head lower down so you don't have to push for as long. You may already feel a strong urge to push, and you may not be able to stop yourself as the feeling can become overwhelming! On the other hand, you may not feel an urge to push if you have an epidural. In that case, your medical team will help to encourage you to push in coordination with contractions to maximise effectiveness in moving the baby downward.

You can choose different positions for pushing, including lying on your back, squatting, kneeling, or using a birthing stool or bar depending on what is comfortable for you. This stage can take from 30 minutes up to an hour. As you push with each contraction, the baby gradually descends through the birth canal, until eventually it is visible at the entrance to the vagina, known as the perineum. Your medical team may place their hands around the baby's head, to support your perineum and prevent tearing while ensuring a controlled delivery.

Third stage – delivery of the placenta

After the baby is born, your uterus will continue to contract to expel the placenta, which provided nutrients and oxygen to the baby during pregnancy. Your healthcare provider may gently pull downwards on the umbilical cord, or instruct you to push lightly to aid in the delivery of the placenta. You may also receive an injection to encourage the release of the placenta and reduce the risk of excessive bleeding.

The placenta is usually delivered within 5–30 minutes after the birth of the baby. It will be examined after birth to ensure it is intact and that no fragments are left behind in the uterus, which could lead to complications.

After the delivery of the placenta, the healthcare team will check you and baby for any signs of complications, and provide immediate postpartum care. This may include monitoring vital signs, assessing for bleeding, and supporting you to begin breastfeeding if desired.

Skin-to-skin contact after birth, often called 'kangaroo care', involves placing the newborn directly onto the mother's bare chest or abdomen immediately after delivery. This practice promotes bonding, helps regulate the baby's temperature, breathing, and heart rate, and supports breastfeeding by encouraging the baby's natural rooting reflex.

For caesarean births, or cases where the mother is unable to participate, the partner or another caregiver can often provide skin-to-skin contact. This simple, intimate act offers numerous benefits for both the baby and parent, fostering connection and enhancing the baby's transition to life outside the womb.

DID YOU KNOW?

Delayed cord clamping involves waiting 1–5 minutes after birth before clamping the umbilical cord, allowing extra blood to transfer from the placenta to the baby. This 'placental transfusion' can increase the baby's blood volume and provide an additional 20–30 mg/kg of iron, enough to support their needs for about 3 months. This is especially beneficial for preterm babies, helping stabilise their blood pressure and reduce the risk of iron deficiency, which can impact development.

While generally safe, delayed clamping may slightly increase the risk of jaundice. It can also make it tricky to have early skin-to-skin contact with your baby if you have a short umbilical cord. If there is an ongoing emergency or heavy vaginal bleeding after birth, it may be safer to do immediate cord clamping. Current guidelines from the International Federation of Gynecology and Obstetrics (FIGO), the World Health Organization (WHO), and the UK's National Institute for Health and Care Excellence (NICE) recommend waiting 1–5 minutes for most healthy term births unless immediate clamping is medically necessary.

Instrumental delivery

Having a positive mindset as you approach labour and birth is really valuable. However, a big part of ensuring your overall experience is positive is to ensure you are prepared for the unexpected. Nobody goes into labour hoping to have an instrumental birth, but if you are prepared for all possible ways your birth can go then you can come away with the best experience possible.

Sometimes, instruments can be used to assist the delivery of your baby's head, and these include forceps (which look a bit like salad tongs) or a ventouse (or kiwi) suction cup. These can only be used in the second stage of labour, when you are fully dilated and the baby's head is very low in the birth canal.

There are some situations where they may be recommended:

- **Fetal distress:** If the baby shows signs of distress during labour, such as a slowed heart rate or meconium staining (passage of the baby's first stool), an instrumental birth may be necessary to facilitate a swift delivery and reduce the risk of complications

- **Prolonged labour:** If labour is not progressing efficiently, and you are exhausted, an instrumental birth can expedite the delivery process

- **Maternal health concerns:** If you have certain health conditions, such as heart disease or neurological conditions, healthcare providers may recommend an instrumental birth to minimise risks to the mother and baby

- **Malposition of the baby:** Sometimes, the baby may be in an awkward position, where their head is turned in such a way that it is preventing it from passing through the vaginal canal. In such cases, instruments can be used to help rotate the baby's position and help to deliver the baby

- **Maternal choice:** In some cases, you may wish to request an instrumental birth if you feel unable to continue pushing or if you want to expedite the delivery process for personal reasons

Ventouse and forceps are both safe and effective. Your doctor will choose the type of instrument most suitable for you, your baby, and your situation. There are different types of ventouse and forceps, some of which are specifically designed to turn the baby around, if needed. There are certain factors which may favour one instrument over another, and your doctor can guide you through which is recommended in your specific situation.

Your medical team should talk you through the benefits and risks of the procedure, and gain your consent before proceeding. Generally, an episiotomy (a cut to the perineum) may be recommended to create extra space to help the delivery and reduce the risk of severe tears occurring.

Caesarean birth

A caesarean section (C-section) birth is where your baby is delivered via an operation. It is usually performed through a low incision across the tummy, close to your bikini line. The C-section may be described as elective, meaning the date is planned in advance, or arranged as an emergency procedure.

Even if you have no intention of having a C-section birth, around one in four of all births end in C-section, of which many are arranged as an emergency.[5] Therefore, being prepared and aware of what you can expect can turn what may be a very stressful experience into a more enjoyable one!

Ideas to enhance your C-section experience

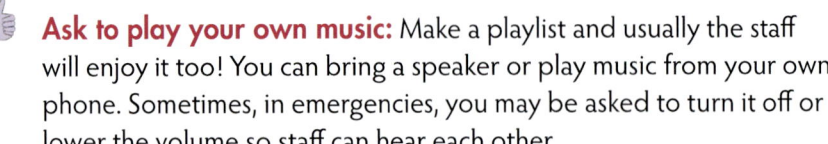

Ask to play your own music: Make a playlist and usually the staff will enjoy it too! You can bring a speaker or play music from your own phone. Sometimes, in emergencies, you may be asked to turn it off or lower the volume so staff can hear each other

Hypnobirthing: Breathing and calming techniques don't just need to be used in labour. By practising these ideas during your C-section, you can relax yourself and separate your mind from the beeping of machines and sickness or discomfort you may be feeling

Ask to drop the drapes: During the operation the sterile drapes will act as a barrier, so you don't need to see what's going on inside. As your baby is delivered, you can ask the doctors to lower the drapes so you and your partner can see the baby as they enter the world. It is best to mention this request before the start of the procedure

Delayed cord clamping: This means waiting for a few minutes after birth before clamping the umbilical cord. Traditionally, it wasn't offered during C-sections because of concerns about mum bleeding. However, we now know that if the procedure is going well and bleeding isn't too heavy, it is beneficial for baby to receive the extra blood by allowing delayed cord clamping (refer back to the box on page 202) for a minute or so. Some doctors may not be comfortable with this during a C-section, or it may not be suitable for you if there is a bleeding risk, so discuss it first

Skin to skin: This is when your baby is put on your chest soon after they are born, so your skin and their skin are in contact. It can be challenging to do this during a C-section because of drapes and machines. Also you are generally lying quite flat so having a baby on your chest can be uncomfortable. However, if your baby is well and you wish to try, your midwife can help you to achieve this even while the operation is ongoing

Who is present during a C-section?

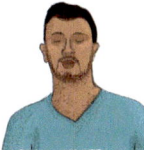

OPERATING DEPARTMENT PRACTITIONER

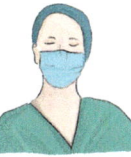

ANAESTHETIST

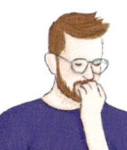

BIRTH PARTNER

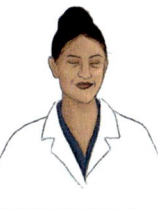

OBSTETRICIAN 1

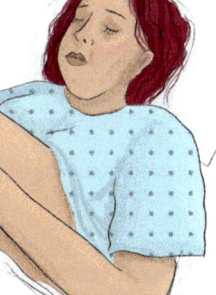

MUM/PREGNANT PERSON

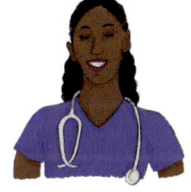

OBSTETRICIAN 2

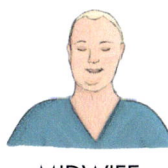

MIDWIFE

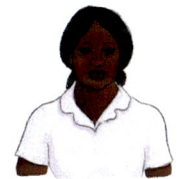

STUDENT MIDWIFE

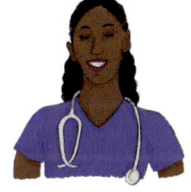

SCRUB NURSE

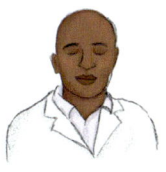

PAEDIATRICIAN

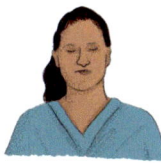

HEALTHCARE ASSISTANT

Postpartum recovery

Although most women have many joyful memories from the early weeks of having a new baby, it can also be a very emotional and overwhelming time. Not only will you be recovering from giving birth and probably not getting much sleep, but you may also be learning to feed, soothe, wash, and change the newest addition to your family.

Amidst all this chaos, it can be hard to find the time to look after yourself and talk about your feelings. Many new mothers struggle with feeling low and/or anxious and it is important to be aware that there are many sources of advice, help, and support.

Some things are great about not being pregnant anymore:

 Almost instantaneous relief on your bladder and not needing to go to the bathroom five times per night

 Not feeling so heavy

 Being able to bend forward to pick something up

 Being able to sleep on your back!

However, there are a lot of changes and challenges to your postpartum body that are much harder to adjust to!

Here is some more about each of those changes and what to expect:

Body shape

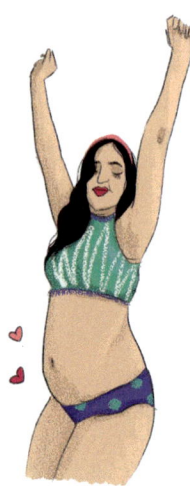

The pressure on women to make their body shape change instantly after the baby is out is immense. Your body has grown a human, after all! In many ways it is unreasonable to ever expect to return to your pre-baby body; partly because some of the changes your body makes the first time you are pregnant, such as the shape of your hips, may actually have changed permanently.

Immediately after birth, your bump will shrink as the baby and extra fluids, like amniotic fluid, are gone. For some, the change is dramatic; for others, more gradual. Over the next few days, uterine involution occurs – your uterus contracts to its original size (about the size of a fist) and returns to its rightful position deep in the pelvis. You will also lose a lot of extra water that you may have been retaining from pregnancy and also the birth process – it can result in some extra trips to pee in the few days after birth.

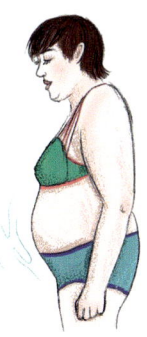

It's normal to feel mild abdominal cramps during this process, especially when breastfeeding, as it helps stimulate uterine contractions.

DID YOU KNOW?

Expect to leave the hospital looking about 6 months pregnant, so pack comfortable, maternity-friendly clothes – not your pre-pregnancy wardrobe! Even after your uterus contracts, you may have some remaining fat and water retention. These reserves supported your baby's growth and pregnancy. Much of it will naturally reduce over time, aided by healthy eating and exercise once you've been cleared. Be patient with yourself – your priorities have shifted dramatically, and fitting in routines with a newborn can be tough. Focus on gradual progress, balancing physical recovery with mental health and confidence. A healthy lifestyle matters, but so does being kind to yourself during this transformative time. You will eventually be able to plan exercise around a routine again, if you want to!

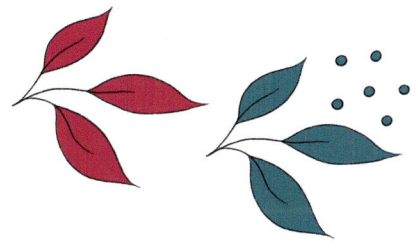

Breasts

Towards the end of the third trimester and immediately after birth, your breasts undergo noticeable changes, whether or not you choose to breast-feed. These include darker nipples, increased breast size, and a feeling of fullness or engorgement. Around days 3–5, your milk typically 'comes in', which can feel uncomfortable or painful. Frozen green cabbage leaves can be placed in your bra to give some relief between feeds!

Breastfeeding works on a supply-and-demand basis: the more the baby latches to the breast, the more signals are sent to your brain to produce more milk, so the milk supply increases in response. The opposite is also true; if you substitute some feeds with bottles, the brain doesn't get a signal from the breasts to produce more milk, so it will reduce the supply as a result. Therefore, certainly in the early newborn period, latch your baby as often as you can, even if they drop off to sleep frequently; small, frequent feeds are fine and help to boost your milk supply.

Pregnancy fashion!

Proper latching is crucial to prevent discomfort and also to maximise milk transfer to the baby. Some nipple discomfort can be expected at the start if you are not used to the feeling of suction. As the baby latches, you may also be aware of a stinging or tingling sensation caused by the 'let-down' reflex, which signals milk flow. While some pain is normal initially, persistent discomfort should be discussed with a midwife, health visitor, or lactation consultant for support.

Bleeding

No matter the type of birth you had (vaginal or caesarean birth), you may experience postpartum vaginal bleeding, known as lochia. This bleeding is typically heavy at first – often heavier than a period – and may increase while nursing before gradually tapering off. For most, it lasts 1–2 weeks but can extend to 4 weeks or longer. If it stops and then restarts, or if you notice clots or bits of tissue in the bleeding, contact your midwife or doctor.

It is better to wear maternity pads or absorbent period underwear, as tampons or menstrual cups should be avoided to prevent infection. The thick maternity pads also have the added benefit of providing cushioning for a sore perineum!

Night sweats

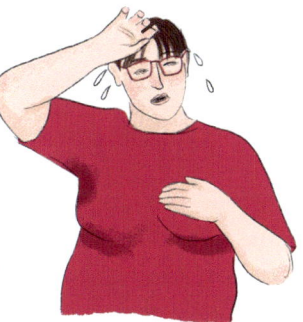

After pregnancy, your oestrogen hormone levels drop, which can cause your body to mimic some of the changes women experience in menopause, including night sweats. If you are also breastfeeding it can supress ovulation and therefore oestrogen levels further, causing the night sweats to last longer than they otherwise would!

For many women the night sweats stop after a few weeks, but they may last longer, up to 6 months, if you breastfeed. During this time, it's really important to stay hydrated and wear lightweight, breathable clothing to sleep in.

Joints

After giving birth, your body undergoes a sudden shift in weight and you will also feel the effect of the joint laxity caused by hormones that prepared your body for childbirth. These changes can lead to joint discomfort in the first few weeks after birth, which may result in back or pelvic pain.

Over time this will settle, but it is important to be cautious with exercise for the first 6 weeks to prevent any undue stress or strain. Staying active during pregnancy will help to ease this change postnatally.

Mental well-being

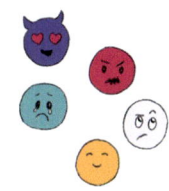

It is extremely important that women feel able to have an open and honest conversation about their mental health during the postpartum period. This is partly because adjusting to parenthood is hard, especially when you are sleep deprived, trying to manage household tasks, looking after other children, and also trying to understand what your baby needs.

But too often women suffer in silence. UK statistics estimate that mental health conditions account for around 10% of deaths of new mothers in the UK in the 6 weeks after having a baby.[6] Mental health conditions are also the leading cause of deaths among UK-based women between 6 weeks and a year following childbirth.

The good news is that with prompt diagnosis and appropriate support and treatment, most people who have developed mental health difficulties make a full recovery.

What are the 'baby blues'?

The baby blues are a very common phenomenon that usually begin in the week following childbirth and can last until a baby is 10 to 14 days old. Women with baby blues can experience low mood and frequent episodes of tearfulness.

It is believed that the baby blues are caused by sudden hormonal and chemical changes after childbirth. As an example: oestrogen levels fall more than 100-fold in the 3 days immediately following baby's delivery.

It is not the same as postnatal depression.

Symptoms of the baby blues

Common symptoms of the baby blues include:

- Low mood
- Anxiety and/or restlessness
- Feeling irritable, touchy, or grumpy
- Recurrent and/or sudden crying spells (including bursting into tears) without any clear cause
- Feeling emotional and/or overwhelmed

While these symptoms might be distressing – particularly at a time where you likely expected to feel very happy – they are normal and do not require medical attention.

The baby blues are a common part of the postpartum experience and, unfortunately, there are no specific treatments available. However, the good news is that, for most new mothers, the symptoms are mild and will pass in a few days.

210

Some helpful tips include:

- Talking about your feelings with your partner, a close friend, or family member

- Try journaling your thoughts and emotions in a notebook

- Ask those close to you for help with tasks around the house (e.g., cleaning, cooking meals, or gardening). It is not easy to ask for help, but remember that this is a very temporary time, and involves massive upheaval in your life. Managing day-to-day tasks on top of everything can feel overwhelming

- It can be helpful to think about the tasks that can be outsourced for a few days/weeks to take some of the pressure off, and consider if you have the resources for someone to help with cleaning, meal delivery/meal prep boxes, childcare for other children

- Pause to take a few deep breaths when you are feeling low, overwhelmed, or tearful. Hypnobirthing or mindfulness techniques can be a practical way to focus your thoughts. Have a look at some apps you can download, like Calm and Headspace

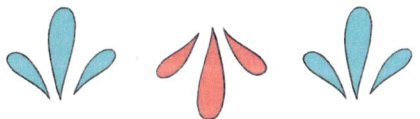

What is postpartum depression?

Postpartum (or postnatal) depression is a type of depressive illness that develops after having a baby. The symptoms are similar to that of depression that develops outside of childbirth, with low mood often being the main complaint.

Postpartum depression can impact on a new mother's ability to take care of herself and her baby. It can make simple, everyday tasks (including childcare) feel like a struggle. Postpartum depression is common, affecting more than 1 in 10 women within a year of childbirth.[7] The symptoms of postpartum depression usually develop within 2–8 weeks of giving birth, but they can begin up to a year after the birth of a baby.

A smaller proportion of women have depressive symptoms which start during pregnancy and continue after childbirth.

What causes postpartum depression?

Postpartum depression often results from a combination of factors rather than a single cause. Evidence suggests that it is more likely to occur in women with a history of mental health issues, depression, or anxiety during pregnancy, recent life stresses (e.g., bereavement or relationship difficulties), or poor social support.[8] Factors like domestic abuse can also increase risk and, in some cases, it may be linked to treatable medical conditions like low vitamin B12 or thyroid issues.

It is important to remember that, for many women, there are no clear causes or contributing factors to their postpartum depression. Also, having experienced one (or more) of the circumstances above does not mean that you will definitely develop postpartum depression.

Symptoms of postpartum depression

Women with postpartum depression can experience one, some, or many of the following symptoms:

Psychological:

- Low mood (e.g., feeling unhappy or tearful for some, most, or all of the time)
- Feeling irritable, hopeless, and/or unable to cope
- Loss of interest in daily tasks and activities (including those you previously enjoyed)
- Poor memory, difficulty concentrating, and/or inability to make decisions
- Loss of interest in sexual intercourse
- Intrusive negative thoughts and/or feelings of guilt
- Anxiety (which can include panic attacks)
- Withdrawing from social contact with other people, including friends and family
- Low self-confidence
- Mood swings, which can range from feeling agitated to apathetic
- Thoughts of self-harm and/or suicide

Physical:

- Changes to your appetite (e.g., loss of appetite or comfort eating)
- Lack of energy and/or feeling excessively tired
- Sleeplessness, meaning difficulty falling or staying asleep, even when you are feeling exhausted
- Aches and pains
- Feeling generally unwell and/or 'not yourself'

Relationship with your baby:

- Difficulty bonding with your baby
- Extreme anxiety about the baby (such as worrying that your baby is unwell or unsafe, even when your baby is well)
- Loss of interest in the baby, which might include feeling apathetic towards your relationship with the baby and/or taking care of the baby
- Concerns that you might harm your baby (either accidentally or intentionally)

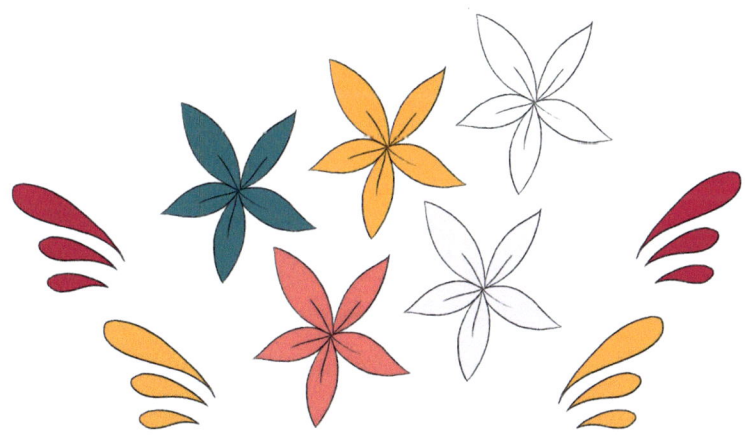

How do I know if I have the baby blues or postpartum depression?

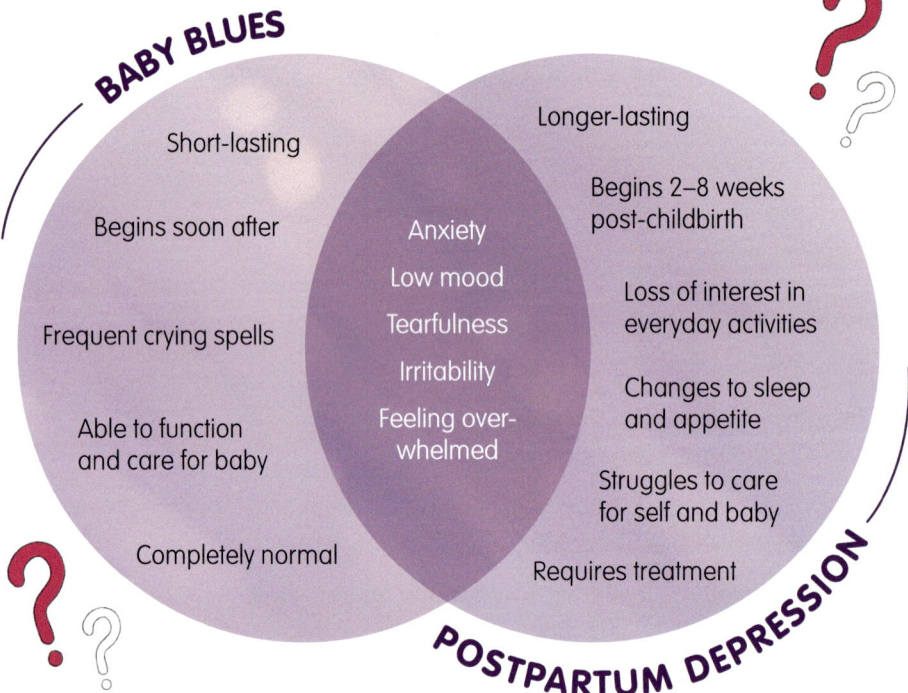

BABY BLUES

Short-lasting

Begins soon after

Frequent crying spells

Able to function and care for baby

Completely normal

Anxiety

Low mood

Tearfulness

Irritability

Feeling over-whelmed

Longer-lasting

Begins 2–8 weeks post-childbirth

Loss of interest in everyday activities

Changes to sleep and appetite

Struggles to care for self and baby

Requires treatment

POSTPARTUM DEPRESSION

The baby blues and postpartum depression have a lot of symptoms in common, including low mood, tearfulness, and irritability. It can sometimes be difficult to tell the two conditions apart. Generally, your symptoms are more likely to be linked with postpartum depression if they are:

- Severe
- Lasting for longer than 2 weeks
- Interfering with your ability to function (e.g., eat and sleep)
- Interfering with your ability to bond with and/or take care of your baby

The only person who can safely and appropriately diagnose your symptoms is a healthcare professional. If you think that you might have postpartum depression (or have any symptoms of concern), it is important that you contact your local health professional promptly to arrange a consultation.

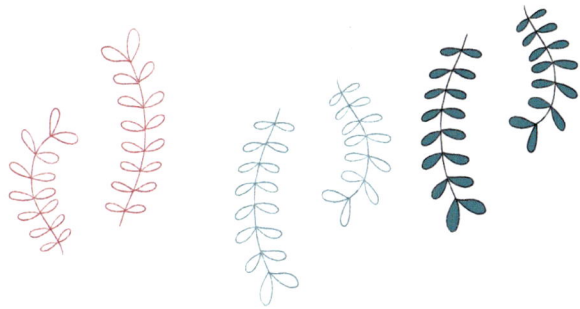

That rounds off our whistle-stop tour of pregnancy and what you can expect. Pregnancy is a time of transformation, not just physically but emotionally, as you prepare to open a new chapter in your life. While the journey may feel overwhelming at times, taking things one day at a time can help it feel more manageable. Focus on the small milestones, trust your instincts, and give yourself space as you adapt to each phase. Remember, every pregnancy is unique, and embracing the experience at your own pace can make it a little less daunting and much more special.

Different types of pregnancy loss

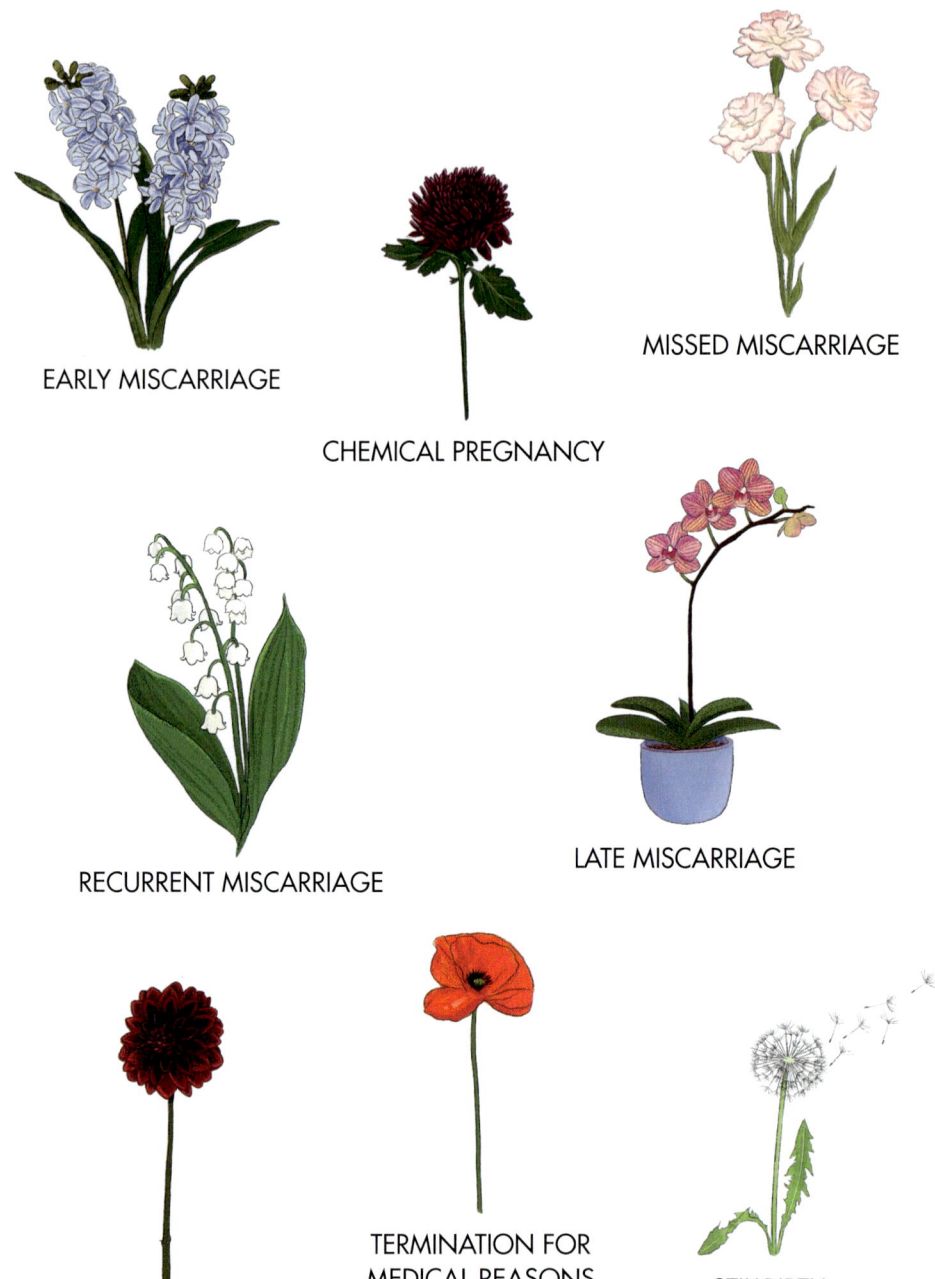

EARLY MISCARRIAGE

CHEMICAL PREGNANCY

MISSED MISCARRIAGE

RECURRENT MISCARRIAGE

LATE MISCARRIAGE

ECTOPIC PREGNANCY

TERMINATION FOR
MEDICAL REASONS

STILLBIRTH

CHAPTER 8

Pregnancy loss

Experiencing any type of pregnancy loss is devastating and can leave you and your partner questioning why it has happened to you. Around the world, there are an estimated 23 million miscarriages every year,[1] yet there is still a lot we don't know about why they happen.

The statistic that 10–20% of all pregnancies ends in miscarriage is widely recognised and cited by numerous organisations and research studies. However, this can often feel like an underestimation, because nothing seems to bring women together like disclosing a pregnancy loss; you quickly realise that many people around you have sadly been through it too, often in silence.

Knowing it is common doesn't necessarily help, but it can help you to feel less alone.

What is a miscarriage?

A miscarriage is the loss of a pregnancy during the first 24 weeks.

Depending on when a miscarriage occurs it can be classified further into:

- **Early miscarriage:** This happens during the first 3 months of pregnancy and is sometimes called a first-trimester miscarriage
- **Late miscarriage:** This happens between 12 and 24 weeks of pregnancy and is sometimes called a second-trimester miscarriage

- **Recurrent miscarriage:** This is the loss of three or more consecutive pregnancies before 24 weeks. This affects approximately 1–2% of couples

- **Missed (silent) miscarriage:** This term refers to when your baby has stopped developing, but there are no immediate signs, such as pain or bleeding. It may only be identified when you attend for your first scan

- **Incomplete miscarriage:** This happens when a miscarriage begins, with signs such as bleeding, but some of your baby's remains or other pregnancy tissue can still be seen in the womb

- **Chemical pregnancy:** This is a term used to describe a very early miscarriage that happens within the first 5 weeks of pregnancy. You may only realise it has happened because your period came a few days later than expected, or you had a positive pregnancy test followed by bleeding

Late pregnancy loss

While the majority of miscarriages take place early in pregnancy, before 12 weeks, unfortunately it is possible to have a miscarriage at any point before birth. If this pregnancy loss occurs after 24 weeks, it is described as a stillbirth. Not only does this tragic event have emotional and psychological consequences, but it is also practically different to manage.

Was it somehow your fault?

When the team looking after you during your pregnancy are unable to give a reason why your miscarriage has happened, it can be really difficult to come to terms with.

Important fact: Miscarriages are rarely caused by something you did or didn't do. Blaming yourself can add unnecessary emotional pain to an already difficult experience.

While we recommend making certain lifestyle changes when you find out you are pregnant, like avoiding alcohol or smoking to reduce the risk of miscarriage, many miscarriages occur even when everything is done 'right'. Even if a behaviour increases the risk, it doesn't mean it caused your miscarriage – most miscarriages happen due to factors beyond anyone's control.

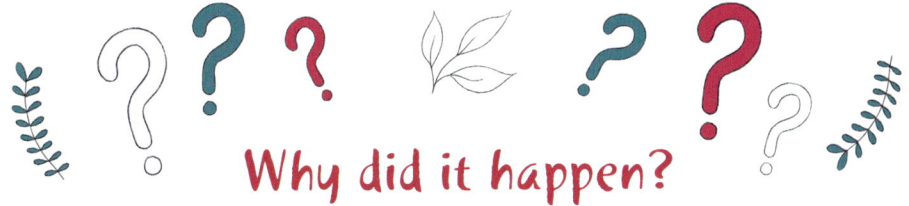

Why did it happen?

One of the hardest parts of being a gynaecologist is not necessarily having an answer to this question. Experiencing a miscarriage is heartbreaking, and the uncertainty of why it happened can make it even harder to process.

For the first or second early miscarriage, you usually won't be offered any tests to understand the exact reason it happened. This can feel frustrating and upsetting when you're seeking closure. The reason for this policy is that most women who have one or two early miscarriages go on to have healthy pregnancies, and further testing may not provide helpful answers.

What we do know is that early miscarriage is most commonly caused by abnormalities in your baby's chromosomes. Chromosomes are thread-like strands in every cell, and they contain instructions for your baby's development. When you get pregnant, your baby gets one copy of chromosomes from the egg and one copy from sperm. When these fuse to create an embryo, something can potentially go wrong, and your baby can get too many or not enough chromosomes. This happens by chance, and if there is an imbalance of chromosomes the pregnancy may be unable to continue and a miscarriage occurs. It isn't because of something you or your partner did or didn't do before or during the pregnancy. It also doesn't necessarily mean that there is anything genetically wrong with either of the parents. Unless it happens multiple times, it is unlikely that these problems could be inherited in the next pregnancy.

Your age

As you get older, it is inevitable that the risk of miscarriage increases because the quality of your eggs decreases. It's important to remember that age only increases the risk of miscarriage and won't always be the cause. Many people over the age of 35 will go on to have healthy and successful pregnancies. (Check out Chapter 5 on fertility for more about age and fertility.)

Medications

Some people may be concerned about whether their medications caused their miscarriage. You may have been taking medications during your pregnancy, either for a pre-existing condition or a new medical concern. Before using any new medication when you are pregnant, it is always best to discuss with your local pharmacist or midwife if it is safe to use during your pregnancy.

Some medications may increase the risk of miscarriage:

- **Non-steroidal anti-inflammatory drugs (NSAIDs)** – such as ibuprofen, which are used for pain and inflammation

- **Retinoids** – used for skin conditions such as acne

- **Methotrexate** – used for autoimmune conditions such as rheumatoid arthritis

If you are using medication that increases the risk of miscarriage, it is always best to let your general practitioner or the team managing your condition know that you are planning a pregnancy. They will be able to discuss the medication and alternatives with you before you start to try for a baby.

If you are planning to try to conceive again after a miscarriage, one medication that is important for you to take is folic acid. This medication can reduce the risk of miscarriage, because it reduces the chance of your baby developing a neural tube defect. It is best to take the folic acid for at least 3 months before falling pregnant to ensure that there are high enough levels in your body when you conceive. If your pregnancy was unexpected, don't panic! You can start taking folic acid as soon as you find out.

Medical conditions

There are certain medical conditions that can increase your risk of having a miscarriage. These include conditions such as antiphospholipid syndrome, thyroid issues, certain infections, or having a weak cervix. While this can be scary, it's important to remember that the team looking after you during your pregnancy will be experienced in managing these conditions and will do everything they can to keep you and your baby safe during the pregnancy.

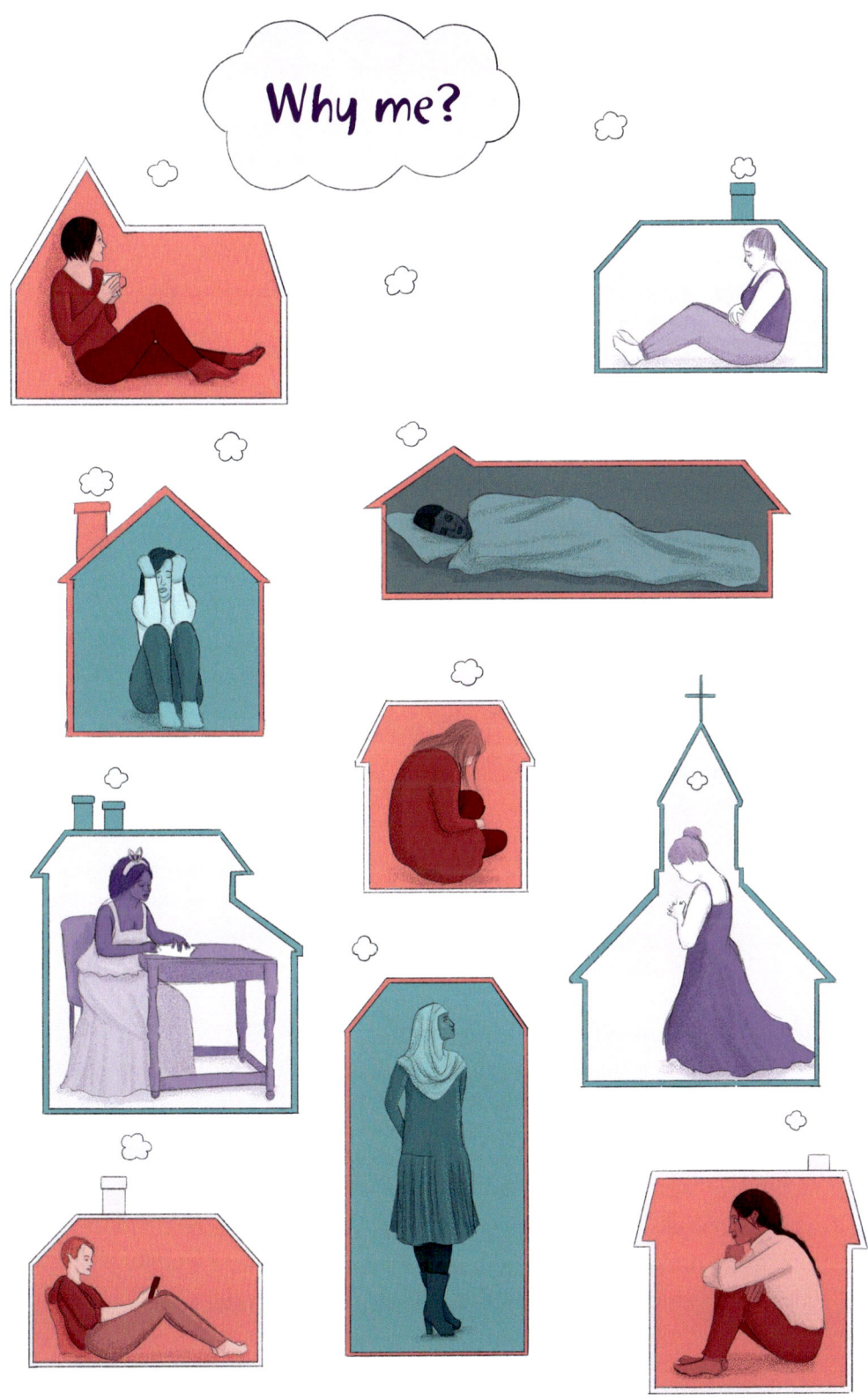

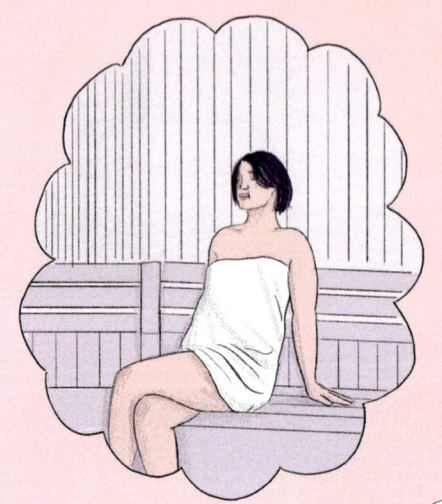

Was it because I used a sauna?

There is no evidence to suggest that occasionally using saunas, jacuzzies, hot tubs, and steam rooms during pregnancy causes miscarriage.

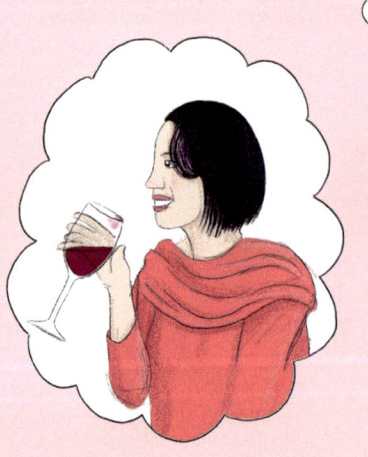

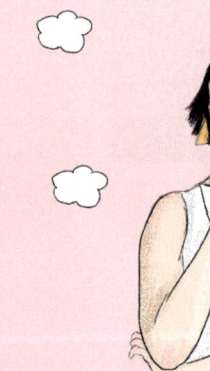

Was it because I drank alcohol early in my pregnancy?

This is very unlikely. If you drank small amounts of alcohol before you realised you were pregnant, the risk of harm to the baby is low. Many women drink alcohol early in their pregnancy because they don't realise they are pregnant and go on to have healthy babies. It is highly unlikely that your miscarriage was caused by a couple of drinks.

222

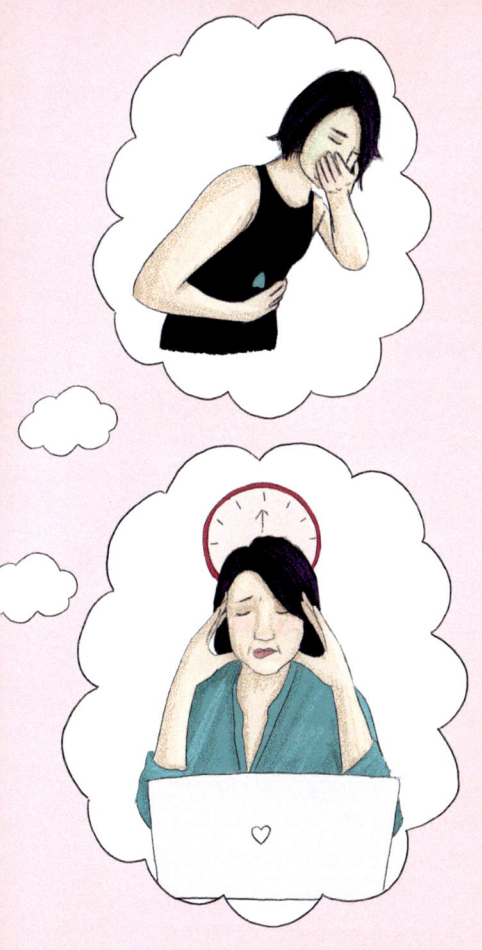

Was it because I ate something wrong?

It is true that food poisoning can slightly increase the risk of miscarriage. However, it's important to remember that even if you have been ill, this does not necessarily mean that your illness caused you to miscarry – it is likely to be a coincidence.

Was it because of stress at work?

It's natural to get a bit stressed in pregnancy, and being concerned about whether anxiety or stress affected your baby is understandable. However, stress is not linked to an increased risk of miscarriage.

It is hoped that, with more research, we will be able to understand why miscarriage happens and become better at preventing it.

If you unfortunately experience three or more miscarriages (recurrent miscarriage) then you should be referred to a specialist who can help to investigate if there is any specific cause for why this is happening to you.

Hopefully one day we will be able to give answers, without having to experience three devastating losses before tests can be arranged.

If you are struggling to cope after a miscarriage, please talk to the team looking after you or your own doctor. They will be able to tell you more about how to access support locally or get a referral.

How will my miscarriage be managed?

When your miscarriage is first diagnosed, it can often come as a shock, although sometimes it may be something you have suspected, but the ultrasound scan confirms it. Sometimes there may be uncertainty because if a pregnancy is very small and the scan is too early, you may have to endure a wait before the miscarriage is confirmed.

For some people, their first wish once a miscarriage has been confirmed is to get the process of managing their miscarriage underway. For others, they may need some time to process the loss before thinking about the next steps.

If you have a missed or incomplete miscarriage, doctors will need to make sure the remains of your baby and pregnancy tissue don't stay in your womb. This is sometimes called management of miscarriage. The doctor or nurse will explain to you a few options available to you. Managing a miscarriage is important in order to prevent complications such as infection or excessive bleeding, provide emotional closure and also to alleviate physical discomfort. By ensuring your uterus is empty, it can allow the body to prepare for future pregnancies.

Here are the options you may be provided with:

1. **Conservative management:** This involves monitoring you closely without any medical or surgical intervention. This approach is often chosen if your body has already begun the process of miscarriage itself by bleeding. It can be an appropriate choice if there are no signs of infection, bleeding is not excessive, and there are no other complica- 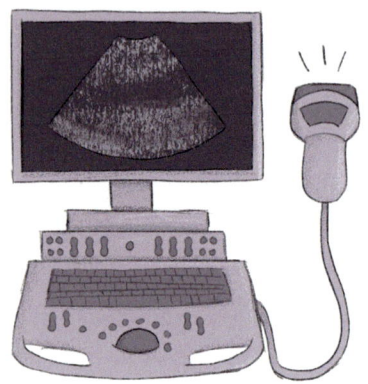 tions. It allows for the body to complete the miscarriage process on its own. The main downside is that it can be unpredictable and, although the process can start, it may sometimes not continue. You will often have repeat scans at intervals of around 2–3 weeks to check if there has been any change. If any of your pregnancy can still be seen within the womb, doctors may suggest one of the next options for management

2. **Medical management:** This option involves the use of medications to help the body to release the pregnancy tissue. The most commonly used medication for this purpose is misoprostol, which is similar to the hormone prostaglandin. It is usually administered by taking tablets orally or placing them directly into the vagina. Misoprostol helps to soften the cervix and bring on contractions of the uterus, helping to expel the remaining tissue. People having a miscarriage 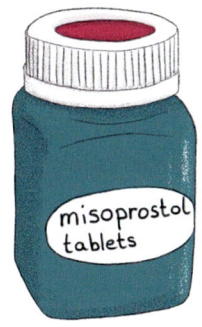 may choose this approach if conservative management has not been successful or if they don't wish to wait for the miscarriage process to start on its own

3. **Surgical management:** Surgical management, also known as dilation and curettage (D&C), or evacuation of retained products of pregnancy (ERPC) is a procedure performed to remove the remaining pregnancy tissue from the uterus. It involves opening the cervix, and then using a suction device or curette to remove the tissue. It is not an operation in the traditional sense as there are no cuts on the abdomen or vagina, but it is still described as a surgery or procedure.

    Surgical management may be recommended in certain situations, like if you have come to the hospital with very heavy bleeding, if conservative or medical managements haven't successfully emptied the uterus, or if there are any signs of infection. It is also an option for women who prefer a more immediate resolution to the miscarriage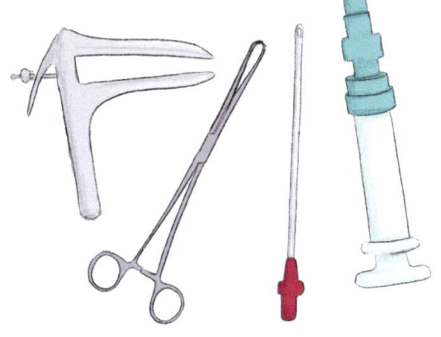

The option which is right for you is a personal choice, and one you should discuss with your medical team. To help you decide, we consider your overall health (both physically and emotionally), the size of the pregnancy or any retained parts of the pregnancy, and if there are any complications such as infections. The team looking after you can help with talking through the pros and cons of each, as well as offering you and your partner support to understand what you can expect.

DID YOU KNOW?

What is a molar pregnancy? This is another type of pregnancy loss (which is less common) and involves a group of conditions known as gestational trophoblastic disease (GTD), otherwise known as a hydatidiform mole. It happens when there is a problem at the time of fertilisation of the egg, for example, if a single egg is fertilised by two sperms as this leads to an imbalance of genetic material. This causes the growth of abnormal cells or clusters of water-filled sacs inside the womb.

Unfortunately, this pregnancy cannot survive, and it is important that the cells from this type of pregnancy are fully removed from the womb. Molar pregnancies are benign (not cancerous) but there is a very small risk that the molar cells could become cancerous if they are not all removed.

What happens next?

Depending on which management option you choose, you will be told how we can confirm the miscarriage process is completed. The completion of a miscarriage can be confirmed by repeating your pregnancy test after 2–3 weeks, or having another ultrasound scan to see that the uterus is empty. At this point you can be comfortable that you won't need any further interventions for this loss.

If you opted for medical or surgical management, there may sometimes be some pregnancy tissue which is sent to the lab to be checked under a microscope. Unfortunately, the results from the analysis of the pregnancy tissue are not able to tell you the cause of the miscarriage. The purpose of this test is to confirm that the pregnancy tissue was normal, rather than showing signs of something called a molar pregnancy.

Once the tests have been completed, you will have the option of deciding what happens next to the pregnancy remains that were examined, and your medical team should be able to talk you through the choices. One option is for the hospital to arrange a sensitive burial or cremation of the remains of your pregnancy. Otherwise, you can arrange your own private burial or cremation.

If your pregnancy ends before 24 weeks, you will not usually need to formally register a miscarriage. However, you may be able to get a certificate in memory of your baby, if you want one.

After a miscarriage

You may experience a range of emotions after having a miscarriage, from sadness to anger and even a feeling of isolation or loneliness. All of these emotions are a difficult but normal part of the grieving process. Ideally, everyone who experiences a miscarriage should be offered support and even therapy to help them come to terms with the loss. Sadly, this is usually not widely available, but you should certainly not suffer in silence. Whether or not professional support is available, many people find talking to a trusted friend or family member can help with their healing.

You may have questions like how long you should take off work or when you can consider trying for another pregnancy. You should feel free to reach out and ask these questions of your gynaecology team, nurse, or your general practitioner.

Emotional impact

Sometimes the emotional impact of a miscarriage is felt immediately, whereas in other cases it can take weeks or even months.

It's common to feel tired, lose your appetite, and have difficulty sleeping after a miscarriage. You may also feel a sense of guilt, shock, sadness, and anger – sometimes at a partner, or at friends or family members who have had successful pregnancies.

Different people grieve in different ways. Some people come to terms with their grief after a few weeks of having a miscarriage and start planning for their next pregnancy. For others, the thought of planning another pregnancy is too traumatic, at least in the short term. Miscarriage can also be the start of anxiety or depression.

If you're in a relationship, it can help to make sure you're both open about how you are feeling. Your partner is also likely to be affected by the loss.

When can I have sex again after a miscarriage?

It is best to avoid having sex until all your miscarriage symptoms, such as bleeding or pain have gone. Your periods should return within 4–8 weeks of your miscarriage, although it may take several months to settle into a regular cycle.

If you do not wish to get pregnant, you should use contraception immediately.

When can I try to conceive again?

If you do want to get pregnant again, you may want to discuss it with your general practitioner or hospital care team. Make sure you are feeling physically and emotionally well before trying for another pregnancy. The advice is usually to wait until you have had a period following the miscarriage before trying again to conceive. The aim is to ensure your womb is empty and there is a fresh uterine lining to reduce the risk of infection. Waiting until you have had your next period also helps with dating the next pregnancy.

Ectopic pregnancy

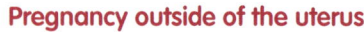

Pregnancy outside of the uterus

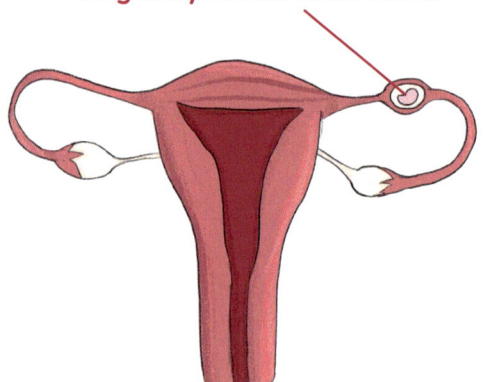

An ectopic pregnancy occurs when a fertilised egg implants and begins to grow outside of the uterus, most commonly in the fallopian tube. Unfortunately, this type of pregnancy will not be viable because the area it has implanted would not be able to supply the blood and nutrients the developing fetus requires. It also cannot be allowed to continue growing as it poses serious risks to the woman's health if left untreated. If the pregnancy became located in a narrow area such as the fallopian tube, it will not be able to accommodate the large size of the growing pregnancy and can potentially burst, causing significant bleeding. Ectopic pregnancies are typically managed through medication or surgery.

Medical management usually involves the use of a medication called methotrexate, which stops the growth of the embryo and allows the body to absorb the pregnancy tissue over time. It is not always the most suitable approach depending on the location and size of the pregnancy, but your own medical team can advise you on your specific situation.

Surgical management is often the recommended approach, where the ectopic pregnancy is removed either by a keyhole or open surgery.

It is important to recognise that ectopic pregnancies are certainly considered a type of pregnancy loss because the embryo cannot develop into a healthy baby. Additionally, the loss of an ectopic pregnancy can be emotionally distressing for the woman and her partner, who are simultaneously dealing with difficult physical consequences of the pregnancy. There are the additional challenges of coping with recovery from surgery, and often the management may involve removal of a fallopian tube, which can have longer-term implications.

Is it possible to still conceive with only one fallopian tube?

Yes! Many studies have actually shown that in the case where an ectopic pregnancy is located in the fallopian tube, there is no long-term difference in fertility outcomes in those people who had a salpingostomy (preservation of fallopian tube) or salpingectomy (removal of one fallopian tube).[2] The reason this is possible may be due to the fact that fallopian tubes can move around, so one fallopian tube can, in fact, move and pick up the eggs released from either ovary at ovulation. It may be reassuring to know there are no 'wasted' cycles; when you ovulate from the ovary with the removed fallopian tube it can still be collected. Pretty cool!

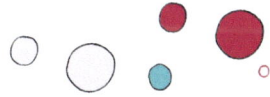

Termination of pregnancy

Termination for medical reasons (TFMR) is also known as medical abortion or therapeutic abortion. This is when a procedure is performed to end a pregnancy due to serious medical complications or fetal abnormalities that would significantly impact the health of the mother or the baby. TFMR is typically managed through medical or surgical interventions, depending on the gestational age of the pregnancy and other factors. Terminations may also be performed for other non-medical reasons like as a result of social circumstances.

Medical management of pregnancy termination involves the use of medications such as mifepristone and misoprostol. This ends the pregnancy and causes the uterus to contract and expel the pregnancy tissue. Surgical management may be necessary in some cases to remove the pregnancy tissue from the uterus, in a procedure that is similar to surgical management of miscarriage.

Despite requiring medical intervention, termination of pregnany is still considered a type of pregnancy loss because it often involves losing a much-wanted pregnancy. The decision to terminate a pregnancy for medical reasons can be emotionally complex and difficult for individuals and their families, often involving grief and mourning.

How to offer support through pregnancy loss

As someone who works in emergency gynaecology units and who meets women going through this on a daily basis, I know that it can be so difficult to know the right thing to say when trying to be helpful in a devastating situation. It's even worse because the vast majority of the time we can't offer comfort by providing a cause or reason to explain what happened.

Many of us will unfortunately experience miscarriage or pregnancy loss personally, or it will affect a close friend or family member. Here are some ideas for what you can do to help in the situation.

While they are going through the process of miscarriage:

- Once you are aware of a loss, acknowledge and say you're sorry
- At an appropriate point, ask her what she needs – but be aware that she may not know immediately.
- Remember to offer the same care and support even if it is not the first loss.
- Offer privacy, support and access to a toilet, and something to wrap around herself if she is bleeding heavily.
- If out in public when the symptoms begin, call a taxi home or to hospital and arrange for someone to go with her, or call her partner.
- You may need to call an ambulance if the bleeding is heavy or she is feeling faint or unwell

For anyone who is going through, or has recently been through a miscarriage, you should:

- Avoid saying phrases beginning with 'at least' such as:

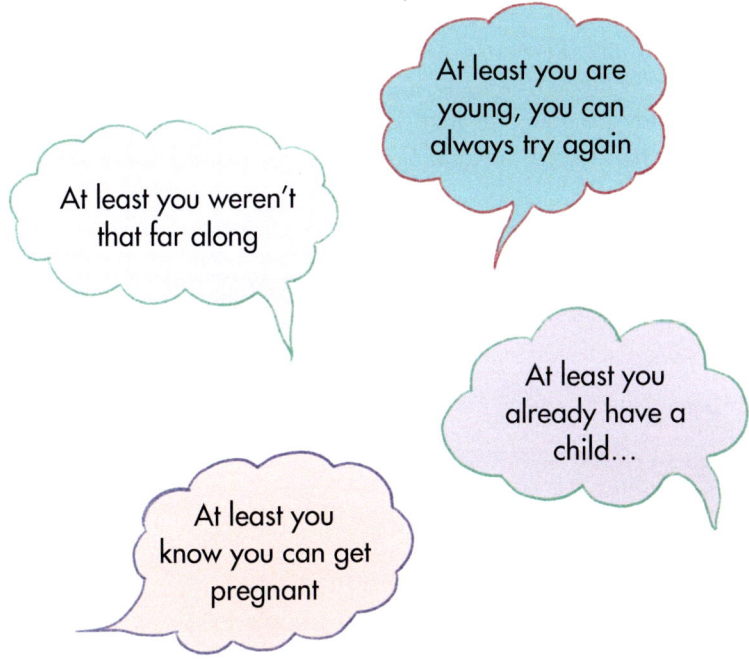

- Avoid using minimising phrases like:

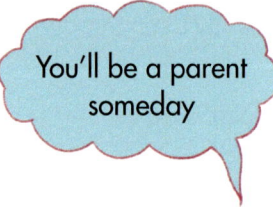

- Avoid making assumptions about future outcomes like:

While you certainly mean well by saying these things, you do not want to minimise what they are going through, or make up answers or meanings behind what has happened. Instead, here are some helpful phrases to say:

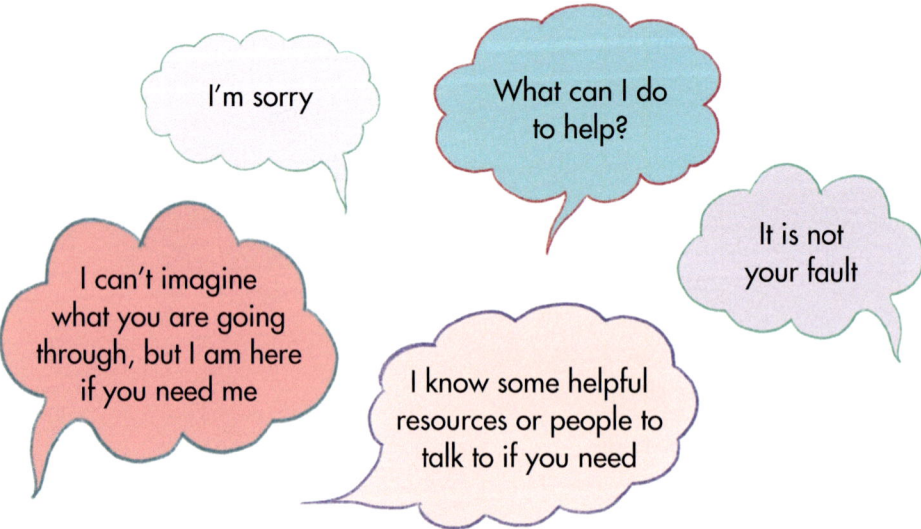

Above all, you can't go wrong by offering help or kind words. When people are in a state of grief, they often struggle to reach out for support, so it's important to be direct and proactive.

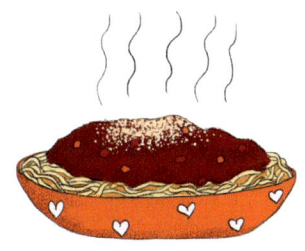

Don't just say, 'Call me if you need anything.' Instead, offer to bring a cooked meal for the next week instead.

Don't be afraid to start conversations; grief can isolate people, so asking how they're doing shows care and love. So many people fear raising the subject of grief and loss in case it triggers upset but instead you can listen without judgement.

Sometimes, the best way to help is by simply being present and letting them share their feelings as they come to terms with the loss and trauma. Recovery starts with talking, so be a great friend or family member and sit and listen.

Pregnancy loss may be a deeply personal and painful experience, but I hope that through the information in this chapter you have found that medical and practical information that can help you to navigate it. Sometimes it can feel like the medical support doesn't go far enough once you are stable from a bleeding perspective, but seeking help at any point – whether from health-care professionals, loved ones, or support groups – can make a meaningful difference. By opening up conversations and breaking the silence around pregnancy loss, I hope we can foster a more compassionate and supportive environment for those affected.

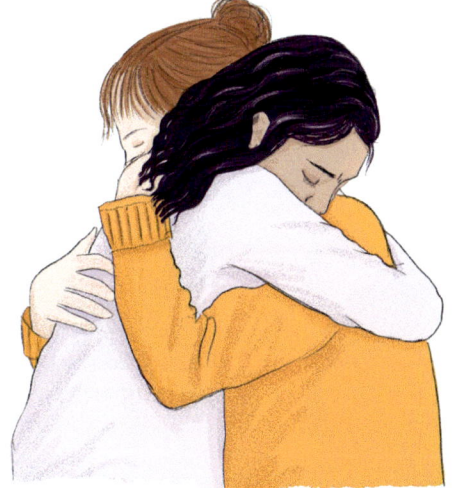

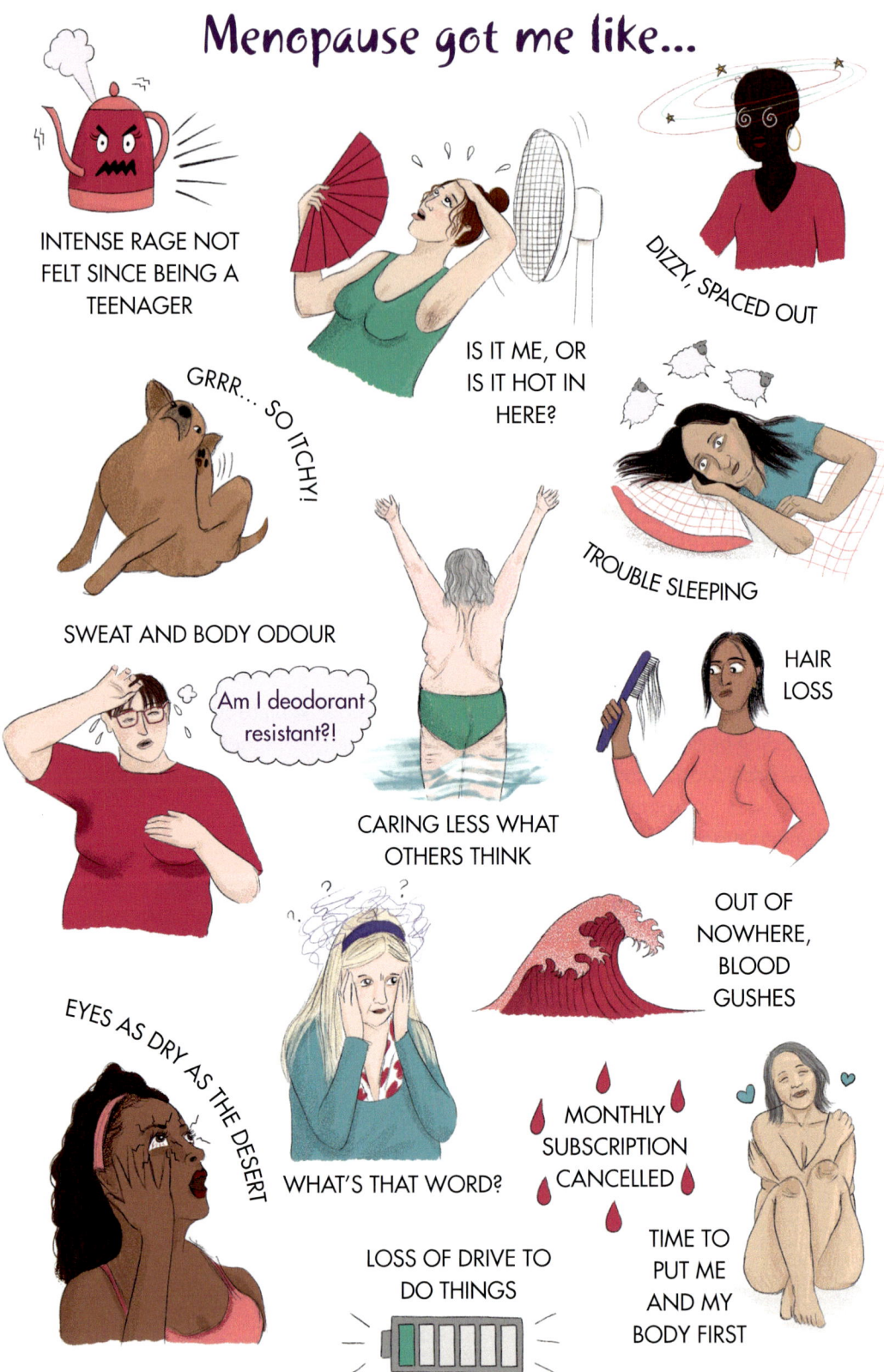

CHAPTER 9

Menopause

Menopause is a natural process that anyone who has periods will experience at some point, but like many other matters affecting women's health, it is often discussed in hushed voices and brushed under the carpet!

Menopause might not be on your radar right now, and it might be quite far away depending on how old you are. However, it's actually very important for everyone to understand, no matter your age!

So, you might be tempted to skip this chapter because it doesn't feel immediately relevant, but I challenge you to read until the end! Here's why we all need to know more about the menopause:

Even if you're not there yet, knowing about menopause can help you to support the women in your life who are going through it, like your mother, aunts, or older colleagues. Plus, understanding it now means you'll be better prepared when your own time comes. Many women, and people with ovaries, aren't fully informed about what to expect during menopause and it can feel like a shock, causing an unexpected impact on your quality of life. Open conversations can ensure that the people who need it can get the right information about the menopause and access support and resources to get these symptoms under control.

By normalising menopause in everyday conversations, we help reduce the isolation that many women feel during this time. It's important for all women and people with ovaries, no matter their background, to feel acknowledged and supported. And it's not just about women; educating men and younger generations about menopause can lead to better understanding and support, improving relationships, and creating more supportive environments at home and work.

What is the menopause?

Menopause is a biological process that marks the end of menstrual cycles. It occurs when the ovaries run out of eggs that are available to be released each month. As a result, the majority of the body's production of oestrogen stops.

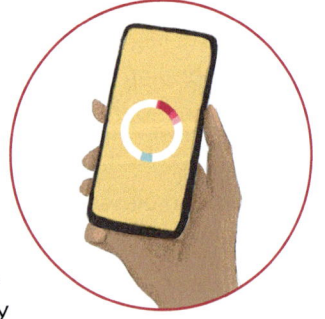

The menopause is officially diagnosed when 12 months have passed without a menstrual period. It usually occurs in women, and people who have ovaries, between the ages of 45 and 55, but it can happen earlier or later.

Here's a breakdown of what happens:

1. **Perimenopause:** This is the transition period leading up to menopause where hormone levels, particularly oestrogen and progesterone, begin to fluctuate and decline. It can last several years and is characterised by changes in menstrual cycles (they can become shorter or longer) and symptoms which occur in response to the drop in oestrogen, such as hot flushes, sleep problems, and mood swings. (Check out Chapter 4 on hormones for more about the roles of oestrogen and progesterone)

DID YOU KNOW?

Did you know just how much women contribute to the economy? Creating supportive environments, especially in the workplace, is vital. Menopausal symptoms can affect work performance but, with the right accommodations, women can stay and continue to work towards their goals, while feeling comfortable to ask for what they need to get there.

The gender health gap refers to the systemic inequalities in healthcare access, research, and treatment that disproportionately affect women, especially in conditions like menopause and endometriosis. According to the World Economic Forum, these conditions can greatly reduce women's quality of life, interfere with their ability to work, and impact their earning potential.For instance, around 80% of women report that menopause negatively affects their daily lives, with up to a third also experiencing depression. Lack of support during this time can result in people quitting their jobs and even leaving the workforce altogether. Endometriosis is similarly linked to missing days off work and affects productivity. Both conditions are vastly underestimated, leading to an underappreciation of their economic impact.[1]

Reducing barriers for women in the workplace could significantly boost economic growth. The International Monetary Fund (IMF) notes that closing the gender gap in the labour force could increase gross domestic product (GDP) by 35%![2] This is a massive figure showing just how important gender inclusion is to the economy. Improving access to healthcare and workplace support for women managing conditions like menopause and endometriosis could lead to an uplift of $130 billion globally by 2040. So, speaking up for yourself and asking for what you need in order to cope and perform better encourages your employers to support not only you, but also other employees and society as a whole.

When workplaces recognise and accommodate the needs of menopausal women, it leads to happier, more productive employees. Implementing concepts like flexible working hours and fostering a culture of empathy can make a huge difference. Progressive employers who openly support menopausal women are more likely to attract and retain talent, which is great for everyone.

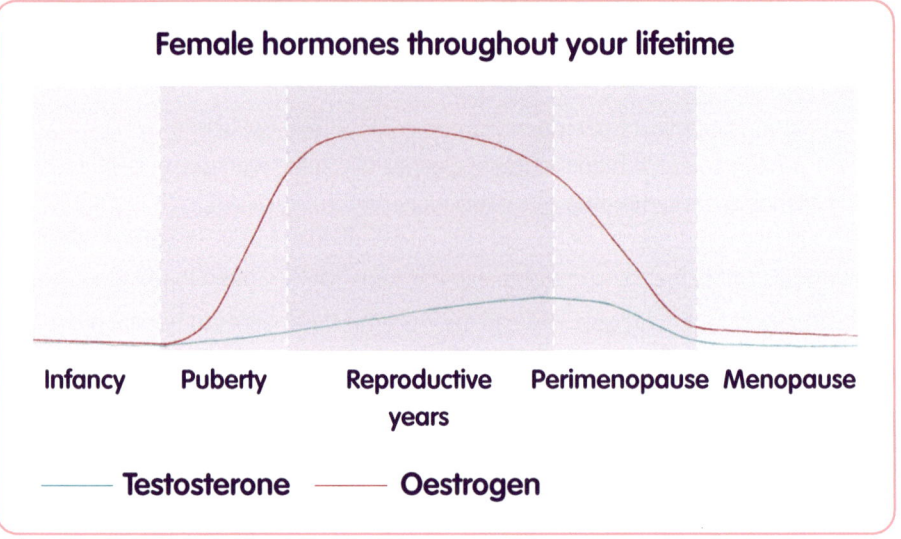

Female hormones throughout your lifetime

Infancy Puberty Reproductive years Perimenopause Menopause

— Testosterone — Oestrogen

2. **Menopause:** This is a single point in time when periods stop permanently. It technically is reached when 12 consecutive months have passed without having a menstrual period. By this time, the ovaries have stopped releasing eggs, and the production of oestrogen and progesterone decreases significantly

3. **Post-menopause:** This is the time of life after menopause has occurred. As the body becomes accustomed to lower levels of oestrogen, symptoms like hot flushes tend to ease off. However, it is important to be aware of the longer-term effects of lower levels of oestrogen as it can lead to other health concerns such as osteoporosis and an increased risk of heart disease

How long do the symptoms of the menopause last?

Some people don't really notice they have entered the perimenopause and only experience very mild or no symptoms. However, for others, the symptoms may go on for some time.

Menopause typically lasts several years, with perimenopause starting around 3–5 years before the definitive menopause occurs. Menopause is confirmed after it has been 12 consecutive months since your last period, and symptoms usually reach a peak around this time. Post-menopausal symptoms can continue for a further 4–5 years, though some women may experience them for longer.

Will a blood test confirm you are in menopause?

Confirming menopause can be tricky, because it usually involves checking the FSH hormone levels. (Check out Chapter 4 for more about FSH!) However, hormones can fluctuate a lot during the perimenopause – one test today might say you are menopausal, but next week it won't.

Instead, menopause is diagnosed when you've gone 12 months without a period. In general, we need to avoid gaslighting women; if you are over the age of 45 and you have symptoms of the perimenopause, then you are most likely in the perimenopause, even though it could be 5 years until your periods fully stop. Your symptoms should be taken seriously and you can have treatment to improve your quality of life.

However, blood tests are useful if you're under 45 with menopause-like symptoms, because this is more unusual, and it is important to rule out other possible causes for the symptoms.

Overall, the entire menopause process can span anywhere from 2 to 15 years.

This can sound scary, but the duration can vary widely between individuals, as do the symptoms. The latter, such as hot flushes, night sweats, and mood changes, can be sporadic and may not be consistent throughout this period. Some people experience symptoms for a shorter duration, while for others, they may continue beyond menopause into post-menopause. Although they may come and go, the intensity and frequency of the symptoms tend to reduce over time.

Premature menopause

Premature menopause, also known as premature ovarian insufficiency (POI), occurs when the ovaries run out of eggs earlier than expected, triggering menopause before the age of 40. This means that periods begin to change, becoming more irregular and unpredictable until they eventually stop, meaning that oestrogen levels drop significantly at a much earlier age than usual.

Premature menopause can occur due to various factors, including genetics, autoimmune diseases, certain medical treatments like chemotherapy or radiation, and sometimes for no identifiable reason (idiopathic).

Someone experiencing premature menopause may experience typical menopausal symptoms such as hot flushes, night sweats, mood changes, and vaginal dryness.

DID YOU KNOW?

In rare cases premature menopause can even occur before puberty begins or has completed, and the lack of oestrogen means puberty can stall or never start.

Because it occurs earlier than usual, POI can have additional impacts as exposure to low oestrogen levels for longer periods of time can increase the risk of osteoporosis and cardiovascular diseases. It can also have significant emotional and psychological effects, due to its impact on fertility.

POI affects fertility as the number and function of eggs in the ovaries declines until they completely run out. While the ovaries may not function regularly, there is still a small chance of spontaneous ovulation – around 5–10% of women with POI can occasionally release an egg and may conceive naturally.[3] For those who cannot ovulate spontaneously but who wish to conceive, assisted reproductive technologies such as IVF using donor eggs may be an option. Adoption and surrogacy also provide pathways to parenthood for those with POI.

As well as the physical impacts, POI brings with it an unexpected recognition that you have moved past a big life stage much earlier than your peers. This recognition can bring with it a sense of loss, and even grief if it was unexpected. Managing POI should involve input from a range of specialists such as hormone doctors who can provide hormone replacement therapy (HRT) to replace the low oestrogen, as well as psychologists and fertility specialists when needed.

What are the symptoms of the menopause?

There are over 30 different symptoms associated with menopause, making it a highly individualised experience. Common symptoms include hot flushes, night sweats, and mood changes, but may also involve joint stiffness, memory problems, sleep disturbances, anxiety, and changes in sex drive, among others. Some people experience no symptoms at all, and others feel like they experience every symptom on the list. Although these experiences are usually described as 'menopausal symptoms', any of these can come on while you are still having periods because the hormone levels gradually decline as menopause approaches.

The intensity and combination of symptoms vary greatly from person to person.

Physical symptoms

- **Changes in periods:** Cycles can become irregular, lighter, or heavier. Some women experience unpredictable periods that significantly disrupt daily life until menstruation stops entirely

- **Hot flushes and night sweats:** Over 80% of women experience these 'vasomotor' symptoms at some point, where sudden heat spreads over the face, neck, and chest, often accompanied by sweating, flushing, and a rapid heartbeat.[4] Night sweats can lead to soaked sheets and disrupted sleep

- **Sleep disturbances:** Trouble falling or staying asleep can arise from hormonal shifts, physical discomfort (like night sweats), or stress. This can worsen feelings of fatigue and irritability

- **Joint and muscle pains:** Aches in joints and muscles are common but often overlooked. Some women also report increased headaches during menopause

- **Vaginal dryness:** With lower oestrogen levels, the vaginal tissues can become thinner and less lubricated, often leading to itching, discomfort, or pain during intimacy. These changes can make sex less enjoyable and may affect both physical and emotional closeness

- **Changes in libido:** The decline in oestrogen and testosterone levels that occur with menopause can reduce sexual desire. This decrease in libido may also be influenced by other symptoms such as vaginal dryness and discomfort during sex. Also, psychological factors like stress, anxiety, and changes in body image during menopause can further impact sexual desire

- **Skin and hair changes:** Declining oestrogen levels can lead to thinner, drier skin, feeling itchy, and hair thinning or loss

- **Other lesser-known symptoms:** There is a whole host of other symptoms of the menopause which don't get as much attention, like tinnitus (ringing in the ears), burning mouth syndrome (a sensation of burning or tingling in the mouth), changes in body odour, dry eyes, increased allergies, electric shock sensations, heart palpitations, and more. These symptoms are less widely recognised but can be just as impactful on daily life

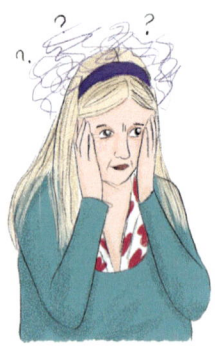

Psychological symptoms

During menopause, several mood-related changes can be noticed, and these are mainly driven by the decline in oestrogen and then can be worsened by sleep disturbances and life stressors. These include mood swings, irritability, or being at an increased risk of depression and anxiety.

Many women going through the menopause are also working, parenting, and caring for relatives, so symptoms such as forgetfulness and poor concentration can have a huge impact. Some people who are particularly struggling with their memory may even mistakenly panic that they are developing dementia, when they are in fact experiencing perimenopausal changes.

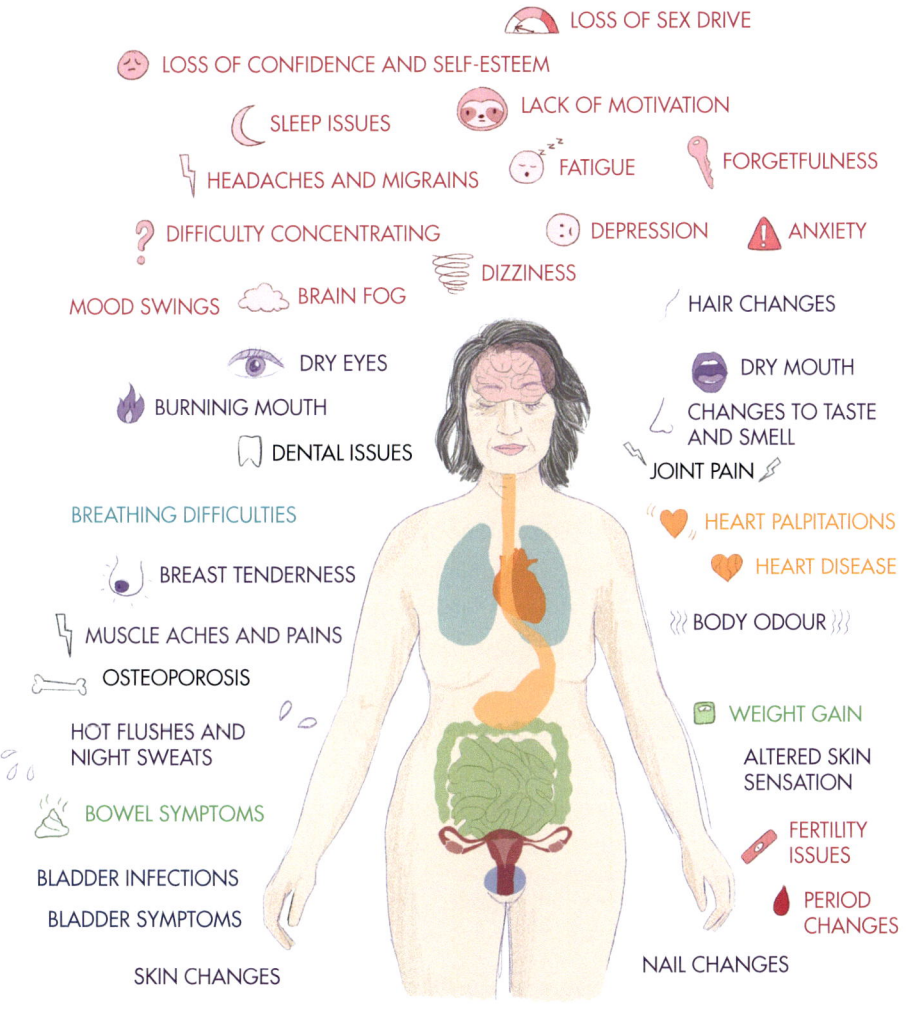

LOSS OF SEX DRIVE

LOSS OF CONFIDENCE AND SELF-ESTEEM

LACK OF MOTIVATION

SLEEP ISSUES

FATIGUE

FORGETFULNESS

HEADACHES AND MIGRAINS

DIFFICULTY CONCENTRATING

DEPRESSION

ANXIETY

DIZZINESS

MOOD SWINGS

BRAIN FOG

HAIR CHANGES

DRY EYES

DRY MOUTH

BURNINIG MOUTH

CHANGES TO TASTE AND SMELL

DENTAL ISSUES

JOINT PAIN

BREATHING DIFFICULTIES

HEART PALPITATIONS

BREAST TENDERNESS

HEART DISEASE

MUSCLE ACHES AND PAINS

BODY ODOUR

OSTEOPOROSIS

WEIGHT GAIN

HOT FLUSHES AND NIGHT SWEATS

ALTERED SKIN SENSATION

BOWEL SYMPTOMS

FERTILITY ISSUES

BLADDER INFECTIONS

PERIOD CHANGES

BLADDER SYMPTOMS

SKIN CHANGES

NAIL CHANGES

VAGINAL DRYNESS, ITCHING, AND IRRITATION

Later-onset symptoms

Some symptoms may be more notable when the low oestrogen levels have been present for longer. This is particularly important in the vagina, because of the effect oestrogen has on supporting vaginal tissues. Vaginal symptoms of the menopause can progress over time, such as needing to pass urine frequently, discomfort passing urine, leaking urine, and having frequent urinary tract infections. These symptoms can be particularly debilitating and distressing.

Is there anything that can help?

Absolutely, there are several ways to manage menopause symptoms, both hormonal and non-hormonal. Managing these symptoms is about finding the right balance and combination of treatments that work for you. An individualised approach is recommended, where the ideal treatment for you is chosen based on your own symptoms and medical history.

Lifestyle changes

Regular exercise, a balanced diet, and good sleep hygiene can significantly improve overall well-being and help manage symptoms like mood swings and sleep disturbances. A mixture of cardiovascular and weight-bearing exercises are suggested as best for bone and heart health.

Exercise and specifically strength training during menopause offers several key benefits, including improved bone density, which helps prevent osteoporosis, and enhanced muscle mass, which supports overall strength and metabolism. Additionally, regular physical activity may help to improve symptoms like mood changes, hot flushes, and weight gain.[5]

Reducing caffeine and alcohol intake, quitting smoking, and staying hydrated can also make a big difference.

Certain supplements are important after the menopause; particularly calcium and vitamin D. This can come from your diet, but some women may benefit from calcium and vitamin D in supplement form to protect their bone health.

Managing sweats and hot flushes

Hot flushes and night sweats are the most common symptoms of the menopause. You may first notice them before your periods completely stop and they can be particularly bad for the first year after the final menstrual period. They may start as an intense heat in the upper body, arms, and face and this can progress to the skin flushing and extreme sweating.

These sweats and flushes are often associated with a feeling of anxiety and a sense of the heart racing. Often, they can happen at night and women may be known to leave their bed to go to an open window to cool off, some needing to change their nightwear due to sweating.

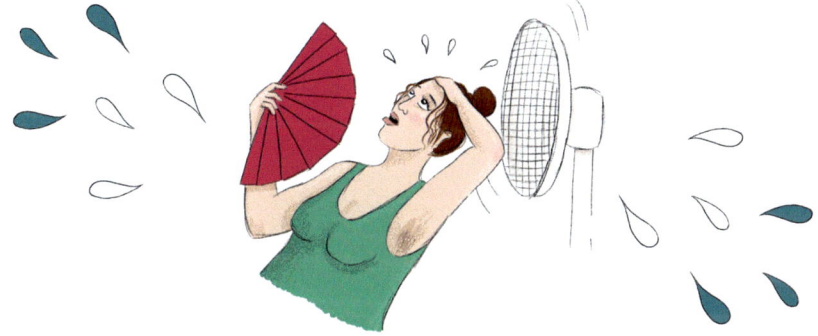

DID YOU KNOW?

'Hot flushes' and 'hot flashes' are the same thing – they both refer to the sudden feeling of heat, often accompanied by sweating and redness, common during menopause. The difference lies in regional language preferences: hot flushes is the term typically used in British English, while hot flashes is more common in American English.

TOP TIPS FOR DEALING WITH THE SUDDEN HEAT:

 AVOID TRIGGERS: You may notice that certain things can trigger flushes like alcohol, caffeine, spicy food, warm temperatures, or even stressful situations. If you can avoid some of these triggers you may even be able to prevent the flush

 THERMAL WATER SPRAYS: These are available in most pharmacies. The water is sprayed as a fine mist onto the face, chest, arms, etc. and can help the skin feel cooler instantly

 WEAR LAYERS: It is helpful to have layers that are easy to put on and take off during the day

 SLEEP IN A COOL ROOM: Try placing a gel cooling pad into your pillowcase or a frozen icepack under the pillow. When you are ready for bed turn the pillow over and lie on the cool side! Another option is to try a satin or silk pillowcase for a similar effect

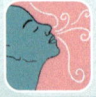 **FOCUS ON BREATHING:** Some people find breathing exercises can help with hot flushes/sweats

Managing psychological symptoms

Cognitive behavioural therapy (CBT) is a treatment for symptoms like anxiety, depression, and sleep disturbances. It helps individuals identify

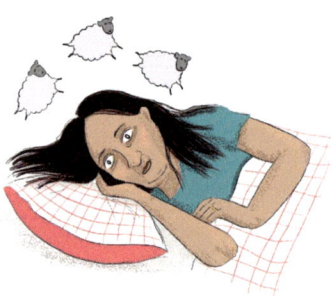 and change negative thought patterns and behaviours, so by developing coping strategies and stress management techniques, CBT can improve overall well-being and quality of life. This can make it easier to handle menopausal changes and reduce the impact of symptoms such as hot flushes, mood swings, and sleep issues.

Managing urinary and sexual issues

When oestrogen levels drop during menopause, it can lead to vaginal dryness, as the body produces less natural lubrication. This can make intimacy uncomfortable, with sensations like dryness, itching, or even burning.

The changes don't stop there. The thinning of vaginal tissues often affects the urethra as well, causing irritation and sensitivity. This might leave you feeling like you need to pee more frequently or urgently. It's a common experience, but support and treatments are available to help manage these symptoms effectively.

Urinary symptoms

Pelvic floor exercises can really help to control some of the urinary symptoms of menopause. Some people use an app to remind them to do these regularly, which may help to prevent future issues. However, if you notice you have symptoms like urinary incontinence that are interfering with everyday life you should not wait for them to improve on their own. Pelvic floor exercises, while beneficial for strengthening the muscles that support the bladder, may not be sufficient alone.

Discuss your main symptoms with a healthcare professional, and you may benefit from working with a women's health physiotherapist, who can provide targeted therapies and exercises, in addition to pelvic floor exercises, to effectively address the full range of symptoms.

Vaginal symptoms

For vaginal dryness, itching, or discomfort, the first treatment to try, usually available over the counter without prescription, is non-hormonal vaginal moisturisers and lubricants. They are useful particularly if the symptoms are mild.

Lubricants should be used before intercourse and can be applied to either partner. There should be no stigma about using it – everyone can benefit from lubricant every time they have sex! Vaginal moisturisers provide longer-term relief and should be applied regularly, typically 2–3 days per week, independent of when you are having intercourse.

Both urinary and vaginal symptoms of the menopause can also benefit from the addition of vaginal oestrogen, but more on that below!

Medications for management of menopausal symptoms

As menopause lowers hormone levels, one effective way to address multiple symptoms simultaneously is by replenishing those hormones through HRT. While HRT has got a bad name in recent years, it can also be incredibly effective and empowering because of just how life-changing the symptoms can be.

Let's take a closer look at the options for hormone treatments for the menopause.

Hormone replacement therapy (HRT)

HRT is the 'gold-standard' treatment as it has been shown to help with a range of menopausal symptoms, and also offers women protection against cardiovascular disease, osteoporosis, and maintenance of muscle mass.

HRT involves replacing hormones that the body no longer produces in adequate amounts. Typically, it involves the replacement of oestrogen, usually alongside progesterone. Oestrogen helps manage symptoms like hot flushes, vaginal dryness, and mood changes, while progesterone is often added to protect the uterine lining in women who have not had a hysterectomy.

In some cases, testosterone replacement might be considered, particularly if a woman is experiencing low libido or other symptoms attributed to decreased testosterone levels. However, it's important to note that the effectiveness of testosterone replacement in women is not as well established as oestrogen and progesterone replacement. Taking external testosterone should be approached with caution due to potential side effects such as acne and hair thinning. The jury is still out as to how effective testosterone is at improving the symptoms it claims to help, and research is still ongoing in this area. You can discuss this option with you own doctor if you are looking for more information.

HRT is highly effective at improving many menopausal symptoms, often providing significant relief for hot flushes, night sweats, vaginal dryness, and mood swings. The impact of starting HRT can be significant for some, as the 'brain fog' starts to lift and you feel like you begin to return to your 'old self' within 3–6 months.

Lived experiences often highlight that HRT can greatly reduce the frequency and intensity of hot flushes, making daily activities more comfortable, and allowing for better sleep. For many, the therapy also improves vaginal dryness and discomfort during intercourse, contributing to a healthier sexual and emotional life. Another benefit is that some people find that HRT helps to stabilise mood swings and anxiety, making it easier to cope with the emotional changes of the menopause.

However, the effectiveness of HRT can vary, and while many find it transformative, others may experience side effects or find that it doesn't fully address their symptoms. It is important to personalise all treatment discussions. All women will experience different severities when it comes to menopausal symptoms – some barely notice any change while others have the full range. Therefore, there is no treatment that is right for everyone.

There are no limits for how long it can be taken for, as long as the HRT is continuing to be necessary and beneficial for symptom control, and improves your quality of life, then you can continue to take it.

Additional potential benefits of HRT:

- Reduced risk of coronary heart disease when oestrogen is started soon after menopause[6]

- Reduced risk of bowel cancer[7]

- Delays or reduces the risk of type 2 diabetes[8]

What are the risks of HRT?

HRT can offer significant benefits, but it also comes with potential risks. Some of the key risks associated with HRT include:

- **Blood clots:** HRT, particularly oral forms, can increase the risk of venous thromboembolism (blood clots) and stroke

- **Heart disease:** There may be an elevated risk of heart disease, especially in women who start HRT 10 years or more after their menopause

- **Endometrial cancer:** This is particularly a concern if someone receives oestrogen-only HRT when they still have a uterus. This risk is significantly reduced by giving progesterone alongside oestrogen

It's crucial for individuals considering HRT to discuss these risks with their healthcare provider to make an informed decision based on their personal health profile and to explore alternative treatments if necessary.

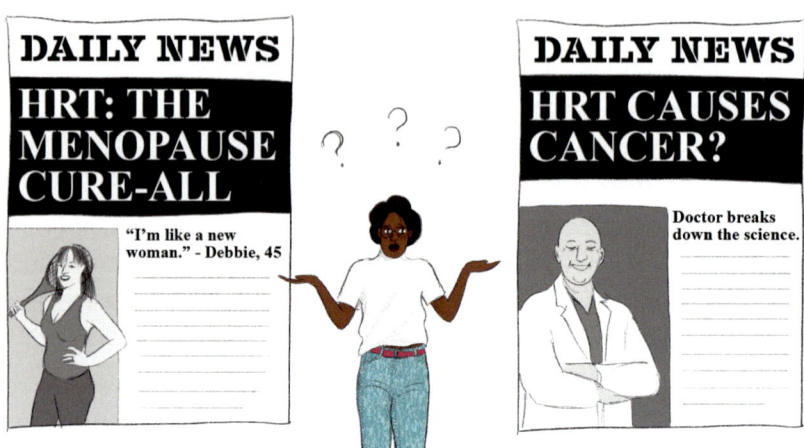

As breast cancer was the focus of concern around HRT, with better evidence we now have extensive guidance which reflects a more nuanced approach to helping decide if HRT should be considered. For most women with a low underlying risk of breast cancer, the benefits of using combined HRT for up to 5 years generally outweigh the potential risks. For them, the symptomatic relief provided by HRT, such as alleviating hot flushes and improving quality of life, surpasses the relatively small risk increase of breast cancer. The amount that the risk of breast cancer increases when you take HRT is typically small. Most women will not develop breast cancer as a result of their HRT use.

Overall, the current advice suggests that long-term use of combined HRT (oestrogen and progesterone) may slightly increase the risk of developing breast cancer – an additional three cases per 1,000 users of combined HRT. While there is an increased risk of breast cancer associated with HRT, it is generally considered small, especially for women who use it for shorter durations or have a low underlying risk.

Oestrogen-only HRT (unopposed oestrogen given without progesterone) can be used in people who have no uterus, or who have previously had a hysterectomy, as they do not require progesterone to protect the endometrium.[10] Evidence also suggests that oestrogen-only HRT actually reduces the risk of breast cancer.

DID YOU KNOW?

How did HRT become so controversial? This began after initial findings from studies like the Women's Health Initiative (WHI) and the Million Women Study published preliminary results that indicated significant risks associated with HRT, including a suggestion that the treatment increased the chances of breast cancer.[9] This led to widespread concern and a significant decline in HRT use globally.

However, subsequent analyses and critiques have questioned some of these findings. For instance, the WHI study primarily involved older women, many of whom had already been in menopause for several years, which may not accurately represent the risk for younger women or those closer to the onset of menopause. Additionally, the type of HRT used in these studies (particularly combined HRT) has been found to carry different risks compared to oestrogen-only HRT.

Further research and longer-term analysis of the same group has suggested that the risks associated with HRT may have been overstated. Instead, it is suggested that when used appropriately, especially in younger women and for shorter durations, the benefits of HRT can outweigh the risks. As a result, guidelines have evolved to recommend a more tailored approach to HRT, emphasising individualised risk assessments and a focus on the short-term management of menopausal symptoms.

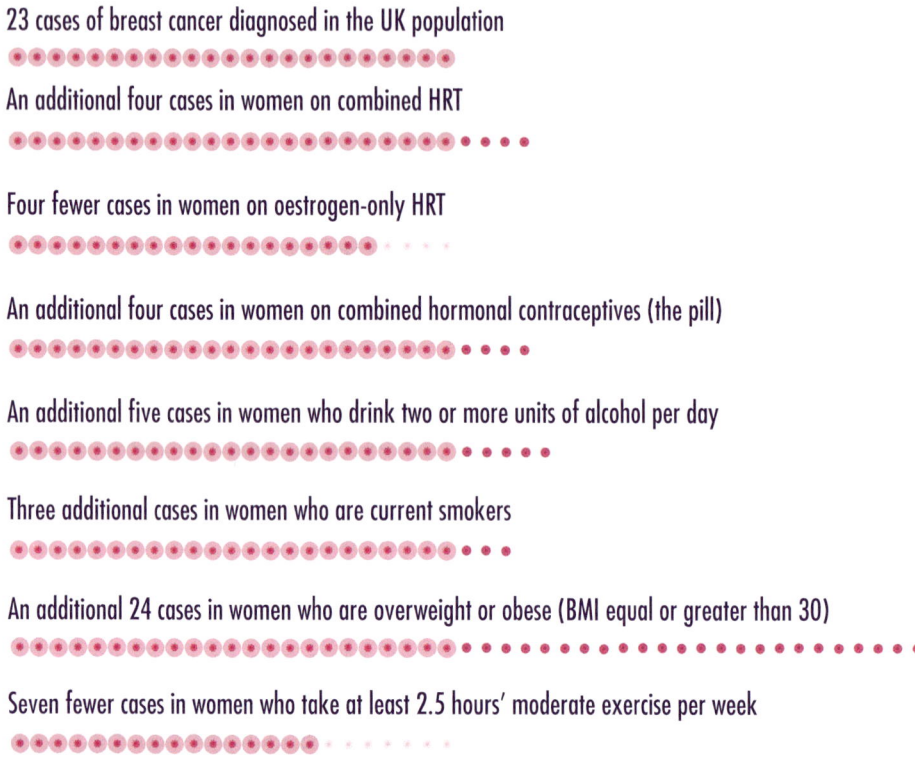

23 cases of breast cancer diagnosed in the UK population

An additional four cases in women on combined HRT

Four fewer cases in women on oestrogen-only HRT

An additional four cases in women on combined hormonal contraceptives (the pill)

An additional five cases in women who drink two or more units of alcohol per day

Three additional cases in women who are current smokers

An additional 24 cases in women who are overweight or obese (BMI equal or greater than 30)

Seven fewer cases in women who take at least 2.5 hours' moderate exercise per week

Data from Women's Health Concern, copyright © 2022 British Menopause Society

Systemic HRT

HRT medications can be administered in various forms such as pills, patches, gels, or creams. It can also be given in a combination of forms depending on the hormones required, where you might have a hormonal coil to provide the progesterone component, in combination with a gel or patch for the oestrogen.

Local oestrogen therapy

When vaginal dryness and discomfort during sex are prominent symptoms, delivering the oestrogen directly to the tissues that require them can be even more effective. Local oestrogen can be given directly into the vagina as creams, tablets, or as part of a ring and is known as topical oestrogen. It can be very effective for specific vaginal symptoms like dryness and irritation, and can be given with or without taking systemic forms of hormone therapy.

Replacing oestrogen in the vagina leads to restoration of the normal vaginal acidic pH, which can increase when oestrogen levels drop in menopause. It can also improve blood flow and can reduce the chances of getting urinary tract infections and overactive bladder symptoms.

If symptoms do not improve with these topical treatments, the next step is to discuss starting systemic HRT such as using the patches/tablets/gels if you are not already using them.

Non-hormonal medications

Some medications originally intended for other conditions, such as antidepressants, can help to manage mood symptoms in menopause. Medications like gabapentin (originally used for nerve pain and seizures) or clonidine (a blood pressure medication) might also be recommended to help reduce hot flushes. This can be particularly helpful if you cannot use or prefer not to use hormone-based therapies.

TOP TIPS FOR SEX AND RELATIONSHIPS AFTER MENOPAUSE:

OPEN COMMUNICATION: Talk openly with your partner about changes in your body and how they affect your sexual relationship. Clear communication can help address concerns and find solutions together

USE LUBRICANTS AND MOISTURISERS: Vaginal dryness is common during menopause. Lubricants can help discomfort during sex, and vaginal moisturisers can provide longer-lasting relief from dryness

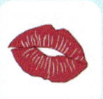

EXPERIMENT WITH DIFFERENT FORMS OF INTIMACY: It can be natural to feel disconnected when your body is changing, and your libido and desire may not be what they once were. Sometimes it can be helpful to remove the focus on penetration as part of intercourse, and prioritise the emotional connection, perhaps with the addition of other forms of intimacy. This includes cuddling, kissing, and mutual massages, which can help enhance emotional connection and physical pleasure

continued...

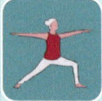 **STAY PHYSICALLY ACTIVE:** Regular exercise can boost libido and improve overall well-being. Activities like yoga can enhance flexibility and help you to connect to your body, as well as promoting mindfulness and reducing stress. This may contribute to a more satisfying sexual experience

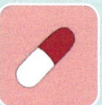 **CONSIDER MEDICAL TREATMENTS:** The symptoms of menopause result from a drop in oestrogen levels, so sometimes the best way to improve the symptoms is by replacing the hormones that are lacking. Consult your healthcare provider about options like local oestrogen therapy or combined systemic hormonal treatments. These can help alleviate symptoms and improve sexual function

 SEEK PROFESSIONAL HELP IF NEEDED: If sexual issues persist, consider talking to a therapist or sex counsellor. They can provide strategies and support to navigate changes during the menopause and enhance communication in your relationship

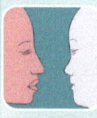 **EDUCATE YOURSELF AND YOUR PARTNER:** Understanding menopause and its effects can help both you and your partner manage expectations and reduce anxiety about changes in your sexual relationship

By addressing these aspects, couples can maintain a healthy and fulfilling sex life after menopause.

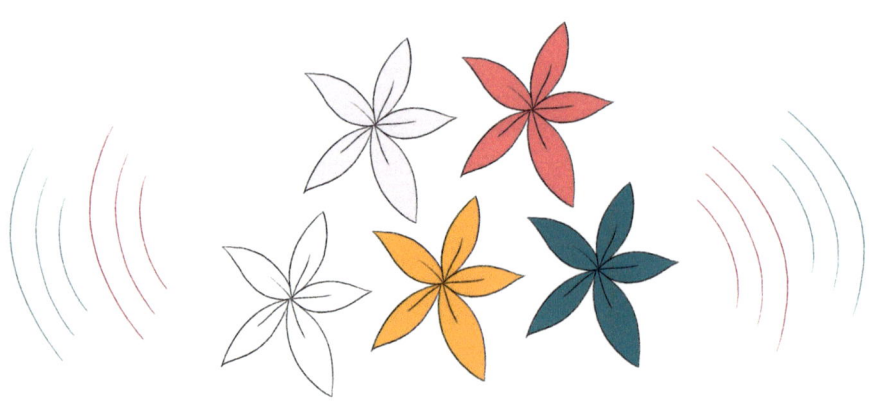

Common misconceptions about menopause

- **Menopause happens suddenly:** Many people believe that menopause occurs abruptly. In reality, menopause is a gradual process that begins with perimenopause, a phase that can last several years before periods stop entirely

- **Menopause only affects older women:** While menopause typically occurs between ages 45 and 55, some women experience it earlier. This may be due to conditions like premature ovarian insufficiency or as a result of medical treatments such as chemotherapy

- **Menopause is just about hot flushes:** Hot flushes are a well-known symptom, but menopause affects many aspects of health, including mood swings, sleep disturbances, concentration, and sexual function

- **HRT is always dangerous:** HRT was widely feared after studies linked it to health risks like breast cancer and heart disease. However, further research has shown that HRT can be safe and effective, especially when started around the time of menopause onset and tailored to your individual health needs

How can you support someone through the menopause?

With so many changes happening at once, going through the perimenopause can feel overwhelming and also isolating. Many people can start to struggle with keeping up with commitments such as family, work and friendships. If you are supporting a friend or colleague going through menopause you can make a huge difference to their well-being and mental health.

Here are some ways to provide support:

Listen and validate

Sometimes, the best support you can offer is a listening ear. Let your friend or colleague share their experiences and feelings without judgement or interruption. Acknowledge that menopause can be challenging. Validating their experiences helps them to feel understood and supported.

Educate yourself

Learn about menopause symptoms and treatments. Understanding what they are going through can help you offer more informed and empathetic support, so that person doesn't feel they have to constantly explain themselves.

Provide practical support

If you're in a position to do so, encourage flexible working arrangements. This could include allowing for breaks, offering remote work options, or adjusting deadlines to accommodate their needs. Sometimes simple practical tools like a desk fan can make a huge difference!

Encourage self-care

Exercise and healthy eating can be a really helpful way of supporting physical and emotional well-being during the menopause, so encouraging or joining them for these activities can be very supportive. Activities like yoga, meditation, and deep-breathing exercises can help manage stress and improve mood.

Be supportive in social settings

Invite them to social activities but be understanding if they need to decline. Menopause symptoms can be unpredictable, and sometimes they might not feel up to socialising. While it's good to offer support, also respect their privacy. Some women may not want to discuss their symptoms in detail.

Encourage seeking professional help

If they're struggling with severe symptoms, suggest they speak to a health-care provider. Professional advice can be crucial for managing menopause effectively.

By offering understanding, practical help, and emotional support, you can make a significant positive impact on the well-being of a friend or colleague going through menopause.

Menopause can bring a mix of challenges, but you don't have to navigate them alone. If symptoms are affecting your well-being, seek advice from a healthcare professional – there are options, from hormone therapy to lifestyle changes, that can help. Prioritise rest, movement, and nutrition, and surround yourself with people who listen and support you. Most importantly, trust yourself – your experience is valid, and you deserve care and understanding through this transition.

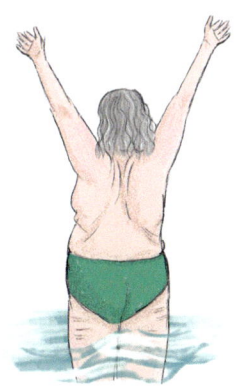

AUTHOR'S NOTE

As you reach the final page of this book, I want to leave you with one key message: knowledge is power, and understanding your body is one of the most valuable things you can do for yourself. When you know what's normal for you, you can recognise changes, ask the right questions, and make decisions with confidence rather than uncertainty. I hope this book has helped answer your questions, sparked curiosity, and encouraged you to pay closer attention to what's normal for you.

This isn't a book you need to absorb all at once. You might find certain sections more relevant at different points in your life, whether it's managing periods, planning a pregnancy, navigating menopause, or just checking in with yourself. Keep coming back to it whenever you need, and let it be a reliable resource whenever questions arise. Your body will change, and so will your needs, but having a solid understanding of how things work will always serve you well. Keep learning, keep asking, and never hesitate to seek answers from a healthcare professional when you need them.

Most importantly, keep the conversation going. Share what you've learned with friends, challenge the stigma around topics that have been brushed aside for too long, and create a culture where people feel safe discussing their health openly. The more we talk, the more we empower ourselves and each other. Thank you for reading, and I hope this book remains a trusted resource whenever you need it.

ACKNOWLEDGEMENTS

No book is created alone, and I am beyond grateful for the people who have helped bring this one to life. First, to my incredible agent, Talia Salomon at InterTalent – thank you for believing in this project from the start and guiding me through this process with such wisdom and support. To my editor, Anna Whiting – your insight, patience, and dedication have been invaluable, and I'm so grateful for the care you've taken to shape this book into what it is. And to Hazel Mead, whose illustrations add so much meaning and clarity – thank you for bringing these ideas to life in such a beautiful and thoughtful way.

To my parents – thank you for teaching me that I can be anything, for instilling in me the confidence to stand by what I believe in, and for encouraging us to try to lead by example. You sacrificed constantly for all of us, and I couldn't be more grateful. To my parents-in-law, Sara and Michael – thank you for welcoming me so warmly into your family, for sharing your son, and for being the most incredible grandparents who step in without hesitation whenever we are both on call. Your love and support mean the world.

To my husband – you are my frame, my rock, my partner in everything, and the funniest, most brilliant speaker in any room. I couldn't ask for a better teammate in life. And to my three wonderful children – Lyla, Coby, and Jonah – you are my greatest inspiration. You give me the drive to fight for a world that is more understanding, more inclusive, and more equal. A world where we uplift those who are different from us, where women can thrive in their careers and be present mothers, and where support, respect, and kindness are at the heart of everything we do. This book is, in part, for you and for the future I hope we can build together.

I also want to extend my gratitude to the many mentors I have had throughout my career – those who have guided me, challenged me, and shaped the doctor I have become. In particular, I want to thank the incredible female gynaecological surgeons who continue to push boundaries and pave the way for those of us following in their footsteps. Your dedication, skill, and determination inspire me every day, and I am proud to be part of this profession because of you.

ENDNOTES

Introduction

1. M. Blackless, A. Charuvastra, A. Derryck, A. Fausto-Sterling, K. Lauzanne, and E. Lee, How sexually dimorphic are we? Review and synthesis. *American Journal of Human Biology*, 2000, 12(2), 151–66. https://doi.org/10.1002/(SICI)1520-6300(200003/04)12:2<151::AID-AJHB1>3.0.CO;2-F

Chapter 1: Getting to know your body

1. P. Charlier, D. Saudamini, and P. Antonio, A brief history of the clitoris. *Archives of Sexual Behavior*, 2020, 49(1), 47–8. https://doi.org/10.1007/s10508-020-01638-6

2. H. E. O'connell, K. V. Sanjeevan, and J. M. Hutson, Anatomy of the clitoris. *Journal of Urology*, 2005, 174(4 Part 1), 1189–95. https://doi.org/10.1097/01.ju.0000173639.38898.cd

Chapter 2: Periods

1. I. S. Fraser, H. O. D. Critchley, M. Broder, and M. G. Munro. The FIGO recommendations on terminologies and definitions for normal and abnormal uterine bleeding. *Seminars in Reproductive Medicine*, 2011, 29(5), 383–90. https://doi.org/10.1055/s-0031-1287662

2. I. S. Fraser, H. O. D. Critchley, M. Broder, and M. G. Munro. The FIGO recommendations on terminologies and definitions for normal and abnormal uterine bleeding. *Seminars in Reproductive Medicine*, 2011, 29(5), 383–90. https://doi.org/10.1055/s-0031-1287662

3. D. Day Baird, D. B. Dunson, M. C. Hill, D. Cousins, and J. M. Schectman. High cumulative incidence of uterine leiomyoma in black and white women: ultrasound evidence. *American Journal of Obstetrics and Gynecology*, 2003, 188(1), 100–7. https://doi.org/10.1067/mob.2003.99

4. European Society of Human Reproduction and Embryology. ESHRE Guideline Endometriosis. Published February 2022. www.eshre.eu/Guidelines-and-Legal/Guidelines/Endometriosis-guideline

5. K. A. Hansen and K. M. Eyster. Genetics and genomics of endometriosis. *Clinical Obstetrics and Gynecology*, 2010, 53(2), 403–12. https://doi.org/10.1097/GRF.0b013e3181db7ca1

6. Revised American Society for Reproductive Medicine classification of endometriosis: 1996. *Fertility and Sterility*, 1997, 67(5), 817–21. https://doi.org/10.1016/s0015-0282(97)81391-x

7. C. Bulletti, M. E. Coccia, S. Battistoni, and A. Borini. Endometriosis and infertility. *Journal of Assisted Reproduction and Genetics*, 2010, 27(8), 441–7. https://doi.org/10.1007/s10815-010-9436-1

Chapter 3: Sex

1. D. A. Frederick, H. K. St. John, J. R. Garcia, and E. A. Lloyd. Differences in orgasm frequency among gay, lesbian, bisexual, and heterosexual men and women in a U.S. national sample. *Archives of Sexual Behavior*, 2018, 47, 273–88. https://doi.org/10.1007/s10508-017-0939-z

2. T. Shirazi, K. J. Renfro, E. Lloyd, and K. Wallen. Women's experience of orgasm during intercourse: question semantics affect women's reports and men's estimates of orgasm occurrence. *Archives of Sexual Behavior*, 2018, 47(3), 605–13. https://doi.org/10.1007/s10508-017-1102-6

3. W. Weijmar Schultz, R. Basson, Y. Binik, D. Eschenbach, U. Wesselmann, and J. Van Lankveld. Women's sexual pain and its management. *Journal of Sexual Medicine*, 2005, 2(3), 301–16. https://doi.org/10.1111/j.1743-6109.2005.20347.x

4. K. R. Mitchell, R. Geary, C. A. Graham, J. Datta, K. Wellings, P. Sonnenberg, et al. Painful sex (dyspareunia) in women: prevalence and associated factors in a British population probability survey. *British Journal of Obstetrics and Gynaecology*, 2017, 124(11), 1689–97. https://doi.org/10.1111/1471-0528.14518

Chapter 4: Hormones

1. K. L. McNulty, K. J. Elliott-Sale, E. Dolan, P. A. Swinton, P. Ansdell, S. Goodall, et al. The effects of menstrual cycle phase on exercise performance in eumenorrheic women: a systematic review and meta-analysis. *Sports Medicine*, 2020, 50(10), 1813–27. https://doi.org/10.1007/s40279-020-01319-3

2. K. F. Michelmore, A. H. Balen, D. B. Dunger, and M. P. Vessey. Polycystic ovaries and associated clinical and biochemical features in young women. *Clinical Endocrinology*, 1999, 51(6), 779–86. https://doi.org/10.1046/j.1365-2265.1999.00886.x

3. G. Bozdag, S. Mumusoglu, D. Zengin, E. Karabulut, and B. O. Yildiz. The prevalence and phenotypic features of polycystic ovary syndrome: a systematic review and meta-analysis. *Human Reproduction*, 2016, 31, 2841–55. https://doi.org/10.1093/humrep/dew218

4. A. E. Joham, R. J. Norman, E. Stener-Victorin, R. S. Legro, S. Franks, L. J. Moran, et al. Polycystic ovary syndrome, *The Lancet Diabetes and Endocrinology*, 2022, 10(9), 668–80. https://doi.org/10.1016/S2213-8587(22)00163-2

5. R. L. Reid and C. N. Soares. Premenstrual dysphoric disorder: contemporary diagnosis and management. *Journal of Obstetrics and Gynaecology Canada*, 2018, 40(2), 215–23. https://doi.org/10.1016/j.jogc.2017.05.018

6. K. A. Yonkers and M. K. Simoni. Premenstrual disorders. *American Journal of Obstetrics and Gynecology*, 2018, 218(1), 68–74. https://doi.org/10.1016/j. ajog.2017.05.045

7. T. J. Reilly, S. Patel, I. C. Unachukwu, C.-L. Knox, C. A. Wilson, M. C. Craig, et al. The prevalence of premenstrual dysphoric disorder: systematic review and meta-analysis. *Journal of Affective Disorders*, 2024, 349, 534–40. https://doi.org/10.1016/j.jad.2024.01.066

8. S. H. Choi and A. Hamidovic. Association between smoking and premenstrual syndrome: a meta-analysis. *Frontiers in Psychiatry*, 2020, 11, 575526. https://doi.org/10.3389/fpsyt.2020.575526

9. Royal College of Obstetricians and Gynaecologists. Managing premenstrual syndrome (PMS). 2018. www.rcog.org.uk/media/mcreb5ix/pi-managing-pre-menstrual-syndrome-pms.pdf

Chapter 5: Fertility

1. United Nations Fund for Population Activities (UNFPA). Seeing the unseen: the case for action in the neglected crisis of unintended pregnancy. 2022. www.unfpa.org/sites/default/files/pub-pdf/EN_SWP22%20report_0.pdf

2. A. Taylor. ABC of subfertility: extent of the problem. *BMJ*, 2003, 327(7412), 434-6. https://doi.org/10.1136/bmj.327.7412.434

3. National Institute for Health and Care Excellence (NICE). Fertility problems: assessment and treatment. Clinical Guideline [CG156]. Published 20 February 2013; last updated 6 September 2017. www.nice.org.uk/guidance/cg156

4. H. Leridon. Can assisted reproduction technology compensate for the natural decline in fertility with age? A model assessment. *Human Reproduction*, 2004. 19(7), 1548–53. https://doi.org/10.1093/humrep/deh304

5. R. H. Goldman, C. Racowsky, L. V. Farland, S. Munné, L. Ribustello, and J. H. Fox. Predicting the likelihood of live birth for elective oocyte cryopreservation: a counseling tool for physicians and patients. *Human Reproduction*, 2017, 32(4), 853–9. https://doi.org/10.1093/humrep/dex008

6. World Health Organization. Infertility prevalence estimates: 1990–2021. www.who.int/publications/i/item/9789200683315

7. R. Wang, N. van Welie, J. van Rijswijk, N. P. Johnson, R. J. Norman, K. Dreyer, et al. (2019), Effectiveness on fertility outcome of tubal flushing with different contrast media: systematic review and network meta-analysis. *Ultrasound in Obstetrics and Gynecology*, 2019, 54, 172–81. https://doi.org/10.1002/uog.20238

8. A. D. A. C. Smith, K. Tilling, S. M. Nelson, and D. A. Lawlor. Live-birth rate associated with repeat in vitro fertilization treatment cycles. *JAMA*, 2015, 314(24), 2654–62. https://doi.org/10.1001/jama.2015.17296

Chapter 6: Contraception

1. Faculty of Sexual and Reproductive Healthcare (FSRH). FSRH Guideline: Contraception for women aged over 40 years. First published August 2017; Amended July 2023. www.fsrh.org/Public/Standards-and-Guidance/Contraception-for-Specific-Populations

2. J. Trussell. Contraceptive failure in the United States. *Contraception*, 2011, 83(5), 397-404. https://doi.org/10.1016/j.contraception.2011.01.021

3. Royal College of Obstetricians and Gynaecologists. Faculty of Sexual & Reproductive Healthcare clinical guidance: management of unscheduled bleeding in women using hormonal contraception. May 2009. www.rcog.org.uk/media/oj5fuf1u/unscheduledbleeding23092009.pdf

4. L. Iversen, S. Sivasubramaniam, A. J. Lee, S. Fielding, and P. C. Hannaford. Lifetime cancer risk and combined oral contraceptives: the Royal College of General Practitioners' Oral Contraception Study. *American Journal of Obstetrics and Gynecology*, 2017, 216(6), 580.e1–580.e9. https://doi.org/10.1016/j.ajog.2017.02.002

5. L. S. Mørch, C. W. Skovlund, P. C. Hannaford, L. Iversen, S. Fielding, and Ø. Lidegaard. Contemporary hormonal contraception and the risk of breast cancer. *New England Journal of Medicine*, 2017, 377(23), 2228–39. https://doi.org/10.1056/NEJMoa1700732

6. American Society for Reproductive Medicine. Combined hormonal contraception and the risk of venous thromboembolism: a guideline. 2016. www.asrm.org/practice-guidance/practice-committee-documents/combined-hormonal-contraception-and-the-risk-of-venous-thromboembolism-a-guideline-2016

7. FSRH. FSRH Clinical Guideline: Fertility awareness methods. Published June 2015. www.fsrh.org/Public/Documents/ceu-guidance-fertility-awareness-methods.aspx

8. J. Trussell. Contraceptive failure in the United States. *Contraception*, 2011, 83(5), 397–404. https://doi.org/10.1016/j.contraception.2011.01.021

9. J. Trussell. Contraceptive failure in the United States. *Contraception*, 2011, 83(5), 397–404. https://doi.org/10.1016/j.contraception.2011.01.021

10. J. T. Jensen, E. Lukkari-Lax, A. Schulze, Y. Wahdan, M. Serrani, and R. Kroll. Contraceptive efficacy and safety of the 52mg levonorgestrel intrauterine system for up to 8 years: findings from the Mirena Extension Trial. *American Journal of Obstetrics and Gynecology*, 2022, 227(6), 873.e1–12. https://doi.org/10.1016/j.ajog.2022.09.007

11. M. Jareid, J. C. Thalabard, M. Aarflot, H. M. Bovelstad, E. Lund, and T. Braaten. Levonorgestrel-releasing intrauterine system use is associated with a decreased risk of ovarian and endometrial cancer, without increased risk of breast cancer: results from the NOWAC study. *Gynecologic Oncology*, 2018, 149, 127–32. https://doi.org/10.1016/j.ygyno.2018.02.006

12. Royal College of Obstetricians and Gynaecologists. Faculty of Sexual & Reproductive Healthcare clinical guidance: management of unscheduled bleeding in women using hormonal contraception. May 2009. www.rcog.org.uk/media/oj5fuf1u/unscheduledbleeding23092009.pdf

Chapter 7: Pregnancy

1. Bumps (Best Use of Medicines in Pregnancy). www.medicinesinpregnancy.org/medicine--pregnancy

2. M. S. Fejzo, J. Trovik, I. J. Grooten, K. Sridharan, T. J. Roseboom, A. Vikanes, et al. Nausea and vomiting of pregnancy and hyperemesis gravidarum. *Nature Reviews Disease Primers*, 2019, 5(1), 62. https://doi.org/10.1038/s41572-019-0110-3

3. American College of Obstetricians and Gynecologists (ACOG). Physical activity and exercise during pregnancy and the postpartum period. ACOG Committee Opinion No. 804. *Obstetrics and Gynecology*, 2020, 135, e178–88. https://doi.org/10.1016/S0140-6736(14)60123-9

4. S. R. Valkenborghs and M. J. Hayman. Physical activity during pregnancy and baby brain development: the elephant in the consulting room. *Neuroscience and Biobehavioral Reviews*, 2024, 159, 105602. https://doi.org/10.1016/j.neubiorev.2024.105602

5. A. P. Betran, J. Ye, A. Moller, A.-B. Moller, J. Paulo Souza, and J. Zhang. Trends and projections of caesarean section rates: global and regional estimates. *BMJ Global Health*, 2021, 6, e005671. https://doi.org/10.1136/bmjgh-2021-005671

6. MBRRACE-UK. Saving lives, improving mothers' care. December 2019. www.npeu.ox.ac.uk/news/1917-mbrrace-uk-release-mbrrace-uk-saving-lives-improving-mothers-care-2

7. N. Khadk, M. J. Fassett, Y. Oyelese, N. A. Mensah, V. Y. Chiu, M. Yeh, M. R. Peltier, et al. Trends in postpartum depression by race/ethnicity and pre-pregnancy body mass index. *JAMA Network Open*, 2024, 7(11), e2446486. https://doi.org/10.1001/jamanetworkopen.2024.46486

8. B. F. Hutchens. Risk factors for postpartum depression: an umbrella review. *Journal of Midwifery and Women's health*, 2020, 22 January. https://doi.org/10.1111/jmwh.13067

Chapter 8: Pregnancy loss

1. S. Quenby, I. D. Gallos, R. K. Dhillon-Smith, M. Podesek, M. D. Stephenson, J. Fisher, et al. Miscarriage matters: the epidemiological, physical, psychological, and economic costs of early pregnancy loss. *The Lancet*, 2021, 397(10285), 1658–67. https://doi.org/10.1016/S0140-6736(21)00682-6

2. F. Mol, N. M. van Mello, A. Strandell, K. Strandell, D. Jurkovic, J. Ross, et al. Salpingotomy versus salpingectomy in women with tubal pregnancy (ESEP study): an open-label, multicentre, randomised controlled trial. *The Lancet*, 2014, 383(9927), 1483–9.

Chapter 9: Menopause

1. World Economic Forum. Closing the women's health gap: a $1 trillion opportunity to improve lives and economies. Insight report. January 2024. www3.weforum.org/docs/WEF_Closing_the_Women%E2%80%99s_Health_Gap_2024.pdf

2. C. Lagarde and J. D. Ostry. Economic gains from gender inclusion: even greater than you thought. International Monetary Fund (IMF) Blogs. 28 November 2018. www.imf.org/en/Blogs/Articles/2018/11/28/blog-economic-gains-from-gender-inclusion-even-greater-than-you-thought

3. British Menopause Society (BMS). Premature ovarian insufficiency: POI. BMS Consensus Statement. April 2024. thebms.org.uk/wp-content/uploads/2024/04/05-BMS-ConsensusStatement-Premature-ovarian-insufficiency-POI-APRIL2024-C.pdf

4. M. Hunter, A. Gentry-Maharaj, A. Ryan, M. Burnell, A. Lanceley, L. Fraser, et al. Prevalence, frequency and problem rating of hot flushes persist in older postmenopausal women: impact of age, body mass index, hysterectomy, hormone therapy use, lifestyle and mood in a cross-sectional cohort study of 10 418 British women aged 54–65. *BJOG: An International Journal of Obstetrics & Gynaecology*, 2012, 119, 40–50.

5. A. Money, A. MacKenzie, G. Norman, C. Eost-Telling, D. Harris, J. McDermott, et al. The impact of physical activity and exercise interventions on symptoms for women experiencing menopause: overview of reviews. *BMC Women's Health*, 2024, 24, 399. https://doi.org/10.1186/s12905-024-03243-4

6. H. N. Hodis and W. J. Mack. Menopausal hormone replacement therapy and reduction of all-cause mortality and cardiovascular disease: it is about time and timing. *The Cancer Journal*, 2022, 28(3), 208–23. https://doi.org/10.1097/PPO.0000000000000591

7. A. Barzi, A. M. Lenz, M. J. Labonte, and H. J. Lenz. Molecular pathways: estrogen pathway in colorectal cancer. *Clinical Cancer Research*, 2013, 19(21), 5842–8. https://doi.org/10.1158/1078-0432.CCR-13-0325

8. F. Mauvais-Jarvis, J. E. Manson, J. C. Stevenson, and V. A. Fonseca. Menopausal hormone therapy and type 2 diabetes prevention: evidence, mechanisms, and clinical implications. *Endocrine Reviews*, 2017, 38(3), 173–88. https://doi.org/10.1210/er.2016-1146

9. J. C. Stevenson and R. D. T. Farmer. HRT and breast cancer: a million women ride again. *Climacteric*, 2020, 23(3), 226–8. https://doi.org/10.1080/13697137.2020.1735797

10. BMS. Fast facts: HRT and breast cancer risk. Tool for Clinicians. November 2022. https://thebms.org.uk/wp-content/uploads/2022/12/12-BMS-TfC-Fast-Facts-HRT-and-Breast-Cancer-Risk-NOV2022-A.pdf

INDEX